HORIZONS IN CLINICAL PHARMACOLOGY

MODERN PHARMACOLOGY-TOXICOLOGY
A Series of Monographs and Textbooks

COORDINATING EDITOR
William F. Bousquet

Division of Biological Research
Searle Laboratories
G. D. Searle & Co.
Chicago, Illinois

ASSOCIATE EDITOR
Roger F. Palmer

University of Miami
School of Medicine
Miami, Florida

Additional Volumes in Preparation

HORIZONS IN
CLINICAL PHARMACOLOGY

Edited by

ROGER F. PALMER

Department of Pharmacology
University of Miami School of Medicine
Miami, Florida

MARCEL DEKKER, INC.   New York and Basel

MARCEL DEKKER, INC.

270 Madison Avenue, New York, New York 10016

LIBRARY OF CONGRESS CATALOG CARD NUMBER: 76-10118

ISBN: 0-8247-6262-2

Current printing (last digit)
10 9 8 7 6 5 4 3 2 1

PRINTED IN THE UNITED STATES OF AMERICA

CONTRIBUTORS

E. De VAUGHN BELTON, Division of Cardio-Renal Drug Products, Food and Drug Administration, Rockville, Maryland

C. PAUL BIANCHI, Department of Pharmacology, University of Pennsylvania School of Medicine, Philadelphia, Pennsylvania

LUTZ BIRNBAUMER, Department of Physiology, Northwestern University School of Medicine, Chicago, Illinois*

ROBERT E. BRUMMETT, Department of Otolaryngology, University of Oregon Health Science Center, Portland, Oregon

ANTHONY H. CASWELL, Department of Pharmacology, University of Miami School of Medicine, Miami, Florida

STEPHEN L. DeFELICE, Clinical Resources, Inc., New York†

KENNETH E. EAKINS, Department of Opthalmology, Columbia University, New York, New York

CARL GRUNFELD, Department of Pharmacology, Albert Einstein College of Medicine, Bronx, New York

GERALD S. LEVEY, Department of Medicine, University of Miami School of Medicine, Miami, Florida

SIMON E. MARKOVICH, Department of Neurology, University of Miami School of Medicine, Miami, Florida††

JOHN M. MARSH, Department of Biochemistry, University of Miami School of Medicine, Miami, Florida

*Present affiliation: Department of Cell Biology, Baylor College of Medicine, Houston, Texas

†Present affiliation: Bio-Basics International, New York, New York

††Currently, Director of EEG Services at Cedars of Lebanon, Mercy, and Pan American Hospitals, Miami, Florida

F. GILBERT McMAHON, Department of Medicine, Tulane University
School of Medicine, New Orleans, Louisiana

JOHN B. MIALE, Department of Pathology, University of Miami School
of Medicine, Miami, Florida

DON H. NICHOLSON, Department of Opthalmology, Bascom Palmer Eye
Institute, University of Miami, Miami, Florida

J. E. PIKE, Experimental Chemistry Department, The Upjohn Company,
Kalamazoo, Michigan

JACK L. RADOMSKI, Department of Pharmacology, University of Miami
School of Medicine, Miami, Florida

HARALD REUTER, Department of Pharmacology, University of Bern,
Bern, Switzerland

ORA MENDELSOHN ROSEN, Departments of Medicine and Molecular Biology,
Albert Einstein College of Medicine, Bronx, New York

ANDREW P. SOMLYO, Pennsylvania Muscle Institute and Departments of
Physiology and Pathology, Presbyterian-University of Pennsylvania
Medical Center, Philadelphia, Pennsylvania

VINCENT A. ZIBOH, Departments of Dermatology and Biochemistry,
University of Miami School of Medicine, Miami, Florida

CONTENTS

HORIZONS IN
CLINICAL PHARMACOLOGY

Chapter 1

INTRODUCTION

Roger F. Palmer

Department of Pharmacology
University of Miami School of Medicine
Miami, Florida

We'd like to welcome you from the University of Miami to the
Second Annual Clinical Pharmacology Symposium. It's gratifying to
see that we have such a good turnout. This symposium is sponsored
by the University of Miami Division of Post Graduate Education,
Department of Pharmacology, in conjunction with the Peninsular
Testing Corporation.

The title of last year's symposium was "New Drugs and New
Developments." Accordingly, we wish to extend the concept of new
drugs and new developments to the problems involved with the first
human dose, problems which are of some concern from both an ethical
and a scientific point of view. Unless these problems are addressed and hopefully solved, they will be stumbling blocks to new
drug development.

A subtitle of this year's symposium is Horizons in Clinical
Pharmacology. I'll reveal my bias; I think that clinical pharmacology cannot ignore basic science. Therefore, two topics were
picked which are important aspects of cellular research, important
to new drug development. They are the isolation of β-adrenergic
receptors and the regulation of cellular control. We will have
concurrent sessions. This afternoon there will be a program on

problems with the first human dose which will be presented under the direction of Dr. Albert Cohen. Simultaneously, Dr. Lincoln Potter will be presiding over a session on the isolation of β-receptors.

Ethical problems with the first human dose regarding who should volunteer, what is the nature of a volunteer, etc., were discussed in great depth, succinctly and completely at the recent Deer Lodge conference with which most of you are familiar. Our emphasis here will be not so much on that aspect as on the science that surrounds the administration of the first human dose. I hope that some agreement can be reached on some of the factors which concern the first human dose. Thus, we have representatives from regulatory agencies, representatives from academia, representatives from the American Society of Pharmacology and, last but not least, representatives from the pharmaceutical industry.

I would like to address myself to academic involvement in the first human dose. Once a drug shows promise from the chemists' shelves, a multitude of data is generated, and finally a clinical investigator is contacted. A series of events then occurs that involves interaction of the investigator with the pharmaceutical company. These interactions concern questions and judgments as to what kinds of data and how much should be generated, what data forms the basis for the amount of the first dose and why. Next, what will be measured after the dose is given? How do we ensure the individual's safety? Must he be normal? Must he be sick? Finally, how can the study be done in the most efficient manner? The answers to these questions are dependent upon the drug in question, the attendant indication for its use, and many other factors which at the present time are too numerous to indicate.

I'd like to take exception to the statement that one of our later speakers, Dr. DeFelice, made that the academic community is still segmented and not fully aware of the principles of drug discovery. I'm sure he didn't mean it to be taken out of context like that, and he'll have a chance to defend himself. But I will

agree with his statement that the judgment of the investigator is
very important in answering the questions posed. In Dr. DeFelice's
book on drug discovery he stated, "Many of the drug developer's
early decisions must be based more on judgment than on fact, no
matter how thoroughly the animal data have been compiled and analyzed." I agree wholeheartedly. But this is precisely the point;
How does one generate the judgment to go ahead with the considerations necessary in the administration of the first human dose?

When we at the University of Miami are approached by industry,
we look at the basic animal data given to us. In the department,
we have at present five clinical pharmacologists and twelve basic
scientists whose interests range from toxicology to very basic biochemistry. We meet and present and discuss the drug in question
with the entire department and review the data presented to us by
the company. Usually a tremendous number of ideas are generated
in terms of how we ought to proceed. Let me give you an example.
A drug in question was being developed as an antihypertensive agent.
However, as we looked at it we saw that its structure had a remote
but significant similarity to quinidine. At this point (indeed in
almost every instance) we wanted to get some of the material ourselves before we gave it to the first human. I can't overemphasize
that principle. It is extremely important to get some of the material. Even when making up a solution of it you may get a feeling
for the way it behaves.

Most faculty have techniques that they trust, e.g., rabbit
atria and intact trained dogs. In other words, we have an entree
into the entire university expertise. Then we perform animal experiments when necessary, and in this particular case we examined
atria and found that the drug did have a negative inotropic effect.
Indeed, it had a negative inotropic effect in the intact dog which
we could dissociate from its hypotensive effect. We examined its
structure and agreed that it would be highly charged, and even
though there were no techniques for measuring its distribution, we
had a pretty good idea how it would be distributed on the basis of

its structure and its resemblance to other compounds. We then com-
municated with the company, asking them for toxicological information, and for other kinds of studies that might be necessary, and
then back and forth again until we were pretty satisfied that we
had a good feeling for what the compound was doing.

We found that therapeutic effects became apparent in the dose
range of 13 to 15 mg when given by rapid infusion in the dog, and
the same in the rabbit atrium. These concentrations would trans-
late into mg/kg by knowing the volume of distribution. Another
kind of information developed from our studies on the Purkinje
fibers was that phase zero depolarization was slowed. Therefore,
we began to look for a widening of the QRS complex in the intact
dog, and we found that the first toxic effect that we could pick up
was not necessarily hypotension or arrhythmias, but we could monitor the fact that the QRS complex was being widened. This would
perhaps be the first sign of toxicity in the human. We found that
the effect of the drug was immediate, but transient, lasting only
30 to 60 seconds when given as a bolus, suggesting again that it
was very rapidly cleared. Other kinds of extremely important information were that Isuprel and norepinephrine rapidly reverse the
toxicity of the drug, giving us a potential antidote.

In addition to the kind of data generated in our own department,
of course, we have an entree as a university-based group to the
entire university system, including the departments of the behavioral sciences, law, and other fields of medicine that we can con-
sult about their different attitudes. We're having some of the
speakers this afternoon speak about some of these attitudes. In
this way, I think we can take all of these resources of the university and bring them to bear on the problem of the first human dose--
what to look for, what to measure, what our ethical considerations
are, and so on.

There are several problems with this approach. Unfortunately,
it may be the least efficient way of developing a new drug. It's
been stated that the Phase I study ought to be "quick and dirty."

Get it over with quick, generate a lot of information, and if somebody gets hurt, well, that's the way it goes. Also, of course, an
academician has other obligations; we can't ask someone to stop in
midstream and take a look at a compound. We've got teaching, patient care, other administrative responsibilities, and currently
we've got crisis committees over training grants and funds and
everything else. As a matter of fact, in the Phase I study that's
currently going on, right in the middle of an intravenous injection
I got a call from the dean to run over to his office immediately
because we had another financial crisis. These are the sorts of
problems that you run into in academia.

I do feel very strongly that one needs a great deal of expertise to give the first dose. It has to be a combination of, at
least in my view, the university and industry, working closely,
trying to understand the problem and bringing to bear all the expertise to finally make a judgment. It's going to be an empiric
judgment ultimately, but it will be the best empiric judgment that
one can make.

Chapter 2

DATA I WOULD LIKE TO SEE

E. De Vaughn Belton

Division of Cardio-Renal Drug Products
Food and Drug Administration
Rockville, Maryland

Let us begin with just a capsule of what the law states. The
law states that a new drug application shall be denied if there is
a lack of substantial evidence that the drug will have the effect
it is represented to have under the conditions of use prescribed,
recommended, or suggested in the proposed labeling. This law goes
on to state that the term adequate evidence means evidence consisting of adequate and well-controlled investigations including clinical investigations by experts qualified by scientific training and
experience to evaluate the effectiveness of the drug involved.
Please note that there's no phraseology in this legislation which
gives status to the testimonial, and that there is a specific requirement for adequate well-controlled clinical trials conducted by
experts. I think it's fair to say that this requirement for efficacy, based upon substantial evidence, in conjunction with our
rapidly expanding knowledge through federal and industry support of
biomedical research, has revolutionized drug development in the
country in the past decade. Today, when a new drug becomes available for use in the care of patients, the physician can have confi-
dence that the major clinical trials supporting efficacy of that
drug have been subjected to critical scrutiny by physicians and

statisticians at the FDA, that the animal toxicology has been carefully reviewed by experienced pharmacologists, that the manufacturer
has been required by our chemists and our inspectors to show that he
can reproducibly produce the marketed dosage form under good manufacturing controls, that a diligent search has been made to identify
the adverse reactions the physician should be familiar with, that
the labeling and packaging of the drug accurately reflect in nonpro-
motional language what is known about the drug and supported by substantial evidence, and that the advertisement of the drug in the
medical literature is under constant surveillance to see that it
conforms with this labeling. That's an all-encompassing statement,
but I want it to lead this presentation because it bears upon the
investigation of new drug procedures.

The scientific staff in our office is about 80 physicians, 40
pharmacologists and 50 chemists. We have other persons doing supporting work in analytical chemistry, pharmacology, toxicology, and
statistics. In the bureau all these people contribute to the ultimate decision regarding the new drug application and the investigational drug application. We currently have about 200 new drug
applications under review and about 3300 active applications for
investigation of new drugs. Many of these are from single investigators, so the actual number of new entities with therapeutic potential is much smaller than this. Thus, the FDA has a team approach
to its review of investigations of new drugs and its ultimate NDA.
I think the critical point here is that the application clearly
identify the significance and safety for the investigational use in
humans. We are going to come back to this a little later.

Let me say just a word about the chemical support of the investigational new drug as we see it going into the first human dose.
Prior to the initial investigational use of new drug substances in
humans, it is required that the preclinical investigations be made
in animals and reports of these investigations be submitted as preliminary presumptive evidence in support of safety and significance
for the proposed use as defined in the investigational application.

Included as an essential part of the preclinical investigation submitted as supportive evidence should be manufacturing control data
which identify and define the new drug substances used in these
studies as the same as those to be incorporated into finished dosage
form and used in the proposed human studies. Our chemist then reviews these materials that come with an investigational application
to certify whether or not significant controls data have been provided for batches of the new drug substance and used in the submitted
preclinical animal studies, including batch identification. For
additional animal studies reported to be made during an investigation,
it should be:

1. Stated whether or not significant controls data have been
   provided for the batches of new drug substances identified
   with the studies
2. Stated whether or not the controls data are essentially the
   same as those reported for batches of new drug substances
   used in the originally submitted preclinical animal studies
3. Stated what those essential differences are such as would
   be involved with the use of different salt forms

Let us turn just a moment to look at another section of the investigational drug application--the pharmacology data. The pharmacology studies should indicate the drug's actions and its rationale
for use, and should include some of the following (let us keep in
mind during the discussion that we're talking about the significance
and safety of the proposed human dose in the proposed human dose):

1. Pharmacodynamic studies--we'd like to see as much as is
   known about the actions of the drug in the initial submission; other data should be submitted as it is generated or
   acquired.
2. Metabolism studies--including absorption, distribution,
   excretion, and comparative biotransformation. Prior to

most testing in humans in Phase I, it is felt that at least
the excretory pattern of the drug should be known. If a
radioactive compound is to be given to humans in Phase I,
studies on absorption, distribution, and excretion may be
appropriate prior to this phase.

Another area is drug interactions. Although we like to see evidence of efficacy in animals, this is not essential if the rationale
for the drug's use is presented. As to toxicology, we have three
different research forms which are ultimately required for new drug
substances--acute toxicity studies, prior to Phase I; subchronic
toxicity studies; and chronic toxicity studies. The duration and
submission of the studies for chronic and subchronic toxicity will
depend upon the duration of intended human use. It may be two weeks
if the drug is to be given only a few times, or it may be six months
or longer. I'd like to go just a little bit into some of this.

We're going to try to divide this up into oral or parenteral
first. If the intended Phase-I study is of several days duration,
the study should have in support of it acute studies of at least two
weeks duration in two species. If it's up to two weeks, we'd like
to see two species, again, for two weeks. If the proposed study is
up to three months, it's two species and four weeks. If it's six
months or longer, two species, three months. Some of the observations we'd like to see during this initial study would be on body
weight, food consumption, and behavior. Hematograms, coagulation
tests, liver- and kidney-function tests, blood-sugar, ophthalmologic
examinations, metabolic studies, and gross and microscopic examinations are also appropriate. For the parenteral preparations particularly, we'd like to see irritation studies and blood compatability
studies where applicable. Now, for inhalation studies, specifically
those concerning general anesthetics, we'd like to see four species
for five days and a dosing of three hours per day. For dermal preparations, with single applications--one species for a single 24-hour
exposure followed by two weeks of observation. For ophthalmic

preparations with single applications--probably one species, and
probably the same as for multiple applications, since we don't usually see a single application. For multiple applications of ophthalmic preparations--one species, three weeks of daily applications as
in clinical use. There are special studies which also might be performed, such as eye irritation studies with graded doses. For vagi-
nal or rectal preparations (multiple applications, again, are usually
the rule)--two species, the duration of application being determined
by the proposed use. For drug combinations (this is not usually the
sort of thing that's done in the initial Phase-I studies, but they
usually come later in a Phase II) we like to see two species for up
to three months.

I want to say just a word to give a complete picture. When
we're talking about contraceptives, estrogens, and progesterones,
our Phase-I studies are usually 90-day studies in rats, dogs, and
monkeys; these are the acute toxicity studies required.

Most of the initial studies are done in males primarily and,
for the most part, they're institutionalized males, whether incar-
cerated in penal institutions or found in medical institutions. If,
after toxicity tests of at least 90 days in rats, there is no indication of antispermatogenic activity, human trials will usually be
allowed. I think that brings in an important point then, perhaps
for later discussion.

I've said very little here about what is required in the use of
children, our so-called therapeutic orphan, or in the initial trials
in women of types of drugs other than oral contraceptives, estrogens,
or progesterones. Now, with respect to carcinogenecity and mutagenecity, we may or may not require these studies. I think the initial application should be accompanied by a diligent search for
compounds similar to the one under study, attempting to find just
how closely related they are and whether or not they themselves have
caused problems in carcinogenecity or mutagenecity. We have no
specific guidelines at this time. However, if we have a reason to
suspect that a compound is mutagenic or carcinogenic, then these

studies may be requested prior to widespread use of the drug. Again, the requirements for oral contraceptives would be different.

Special studies to support the safety or use of the drug, as I've said, would concern such studies as blood-compatibility studies for intravenous preparations, irritation studies for parenterals, eye-irritation studies for ophthalmic solutions, and various studies dictated by the pharmacologic action of the drug. Many of these fields overlap, and what may be required for one area of endeavor, say, dermatologic preparations, would certainly differ greatly from another, such as cardiologic preparations. But again, I think the emphasis is to be put upon the significance of the proposed use.

Now, the purpose of the safety studies in animals is to provide some prediction of the effects which might be expected when the drug is given to man. Animal studies, I think, can alert us to many, but not all, of the difficulties which could be encountered in clinical trials. I suppose it's safe to say that probably the ultimate test of significance and safety of the drug is the human trial. One must remember that studies in animals and humans are usually carried out simultaneously during this initial phase of safety evaluation. Selection of the first human dose should be based upon, we believe, data generated from the previous preclinical studies. The FDA pharmacologists like to see a human safety factor three to five times that of nonrodent species, and about ten times that of a rodent species, just as a general rule of thumb. Other tests or mechanisms for determination of the initial human dose have been proposed, and we could touch on that just for a moment. It has been recommended that perhaps the initial human dose should not be greater than 1/60 of the animal ED 50. Another alternative is that the initial human dose must be considerably less than 1/600 of the lowest LD 50 in any species. Another recommendation has been that the initial human dose should not be greater than 1/50 of the highest tolerated dose in the most sensitive species. For a Phase II--I'm just going to throw this in parenthetically--initial dose usually does not exceed 1/4 of the tolerated dose in the Phase-I study.

I think I've referred already to some of the toxic signs we'd like you to look for, and these are dictated by the preclinical studies.   We would like to see blood level studies, if the methodology is available, and we try to stress these being done as early as possible.   We'd like to see data on half-life accumulation, etc.   Here again, the plea is for early methodology and for definition.

I think one of the things we'd like to see at FDA are pharmacologists and toxicologists and clinicians in FDA working with those in industry and academia to determine an orderly progression of animal studies in relationship to initiation or continuation of the investigation in man.   I'd like to take that a little bit further, and state that we'd like to see a cooperative aspect as far as the continuing clinical trials.   This is not always going to be possible, and it's because of this that I referred to our numbers in the opening remarks. If you're looking at 3300 active INDs, it's not going to be possible to have this type of cooperation on every one.   But what we'd like to do at this point is pick those drugs that we feel have the most promise, or which the industry or academia feels have the most promise (this might also include those which perhaps have a significant degree of hazard), and work together on a proper plan and approach to the study of these drugs.   We'd like to be intimately involved in this process.

Again, I'd like to state that it's most important in this initial planning that we have a clear understanding of goals in approaching the work-up of a drug.   Now I know this changes, perhaps, from day to day, in the course of an investigation.   As new things come to the forefront, the investigational approach will change.

With respect to the recording of data, I'd like to make an important point.   We'd like to see a little more uniformity in the mode of data presentation and the use of the tabulated format.   There have been questions raised within FDA, in informal discussions on this topic, about perhaps grouping together the data which answer a particular question.   If, as I said, the initial design of the study is such that it points out the significance of what is to be gained by the study itself, then certain questions will be raised in the initial work-up of the drug that should be answered in the reports that are forthcoming. I think rather than simply giving a tabulation of results, which is usually done, that you should try to determine, as much as possible, to what extend you have answered the questions that were initially posed.

Some of the other problems that we see, particularly, I think, with single investigators, are problems in formulation of the product. I think this is particularly true where we raise quite a few questions about formulation, chemical controls, etc. which are submitted in the application for investigation (it's the single investigator here I'm talking about). Recently, our bureau director has invited the submission of investigational new drug applications. We tend to usually think of this with respect to those whose drugs cross state lines. But we have been encouraging single investigators, whose drugs are not crossing state lines, to also submit investigational drug applications, because we'd like to be a part of the research and not simply a reviewing effort.

Another problem that we see is the question of drug interactions. Many times people write to us in protocols, indicating that they'd like to put such and such a drug in such and such a fluid and subsequently administer it. So we've raised questions about drug interactions. Adequate animal studies is another area which is giving us some difficulty with single investigators. Here, I think, there's room for improvement in knowledge and its dissemination. Because in many of these cases we know of other studies which relate to the proposed use of the single investigator but are unable to refer him to the data on which we're basing our decision. So I would make a plea here for the early dissemination in the literature of completed studies. I think, however, that we are becoming increasingly adjusted to the cross-dissemination of information in our internal reviews in FDA, and are applying some data that we know of from other studies to new INDs.

Some of the new approaches we might discuss are in the area of

peer review and institutional review committees within universities.
A question along this line has been whether these studies are closely
and critically monitored and assessed or merely rubber stamps. A
proposal has been made to set up some model areas for close cooperation between the FDA and some of the university peer and institutional committees, so that we can clearly define for them our goals and
review procedures. This will enable them, in their own reviews, to
apply the same type of criteria, so that hopefully we would lessen
some of our rereview time. This is an area in which we might move
forward in the next couple of years, with a possibility for certifi-
cation of certain institutional committees. Another area we have
approached is the development of clinical guidelines for classes of
drugs. Many are in the final stages of formulation. These are, of
course, merely guidelines and not formalized protocols. But we hope
that this will aid in the orderly process of clinical investigation,
with protocols to follow.

Yet to be touched upon, I believe, is a significant question
which would be raised early in any protocol. This is the question
of interpreting the final data as it comes in after the study is
complete. I would like to believe that at the time a clinical protocol is initiated, attention would be given as to how the study
will be analyzed, and what the criteria would be for analysis and
effectiveness, notwithstanding that in many instances the criteria
may change, or new criteria may become evident with the passage of
time. We've seen this happen time and time again. I'd like to make
a sincere plea for the investigator's own analysis of his data. I
think this is a critical point.

Touching upon a subject that Dr. Palmer has mentioned, I think
that, because of changing times, the use of investigative subjects
will change. And all the more important, then, is the weighing of
the benefit to be gained against the risk from the investigation itself. In passing, I'd like to toot our horn a little bit because we
have had good cooperation, I think, between FDA and clinical investigators and industry in the areas of peer review and well-controlled

study. There are those who say that a well-controlled study is not
always possible. I'd like to throw out this notion; I just don't
believe that. I believe that well-controlled studies are possible
in all instances. If a study is worth doing, then it's worth doing
properly. Finally, I'd like to harp back again to the IND regula-
tions which require information in support of the significance and
safety in investigation of new drugs in humans. This is a bit different from the new drug application which requires information in
support of efficacy and safety for its proposed use. The key, I
believe, to all of this is the accurate definition of the proposed
study in the human patient, and a clear documentation of the benefit-
to-risk ratio. The posing of postulates and questions to be answered
is paramount. The reports of data should be analyzed in a straight-
forward manner and the answers to questions initially proposed docu-
mented in a clear, concise manner.

Chapter 3

SOME PRACTICAL PROBLEMS IN PHASE I
FROM A CLINICAL INVESTIGATOR'S POINT OF VIEW

F. Gilbert McMahon

Tulane University School of Medicine
New Orleans, Louisiana

The difficulties in extrapolating animal toxicological data, or
for that matter, animal or biochemical efficacy data, to human beings
are tremendous. Historically, governmental regulatory agencies have
required the employment of more and more laboratory animals for longer and longer periods of time. In the 1950's, LD-50s sufficed for
human single-dose studies. If the new drug were to be administered
chronically or subacutely, the animals received several different
doses by the route intended for clinical use, and generally for three
months' duration. For the past five years, the safety evaluation of
new drugs has been largely as reported by Goldenthal in the FDA report of 1968 (Fig. 1). Since then, it appears to me that a relative
stability has been established insofar as the quantitative aspects
of drug toxicity studies are concerned.

The government, the clinical investigator, and the ethical pharmaceutical company are all necessarily concerned with the safety of
the patient. On the other hand, if there is to be therapeutic progress, human research with its intrinsic risks is essential. Not
everyone accepts this today. Primum non nocere is a trite and erroneous slogan which one still hears at medical meetings: "Above all,
do no harm." If this were the primary goal of clinical researchers,

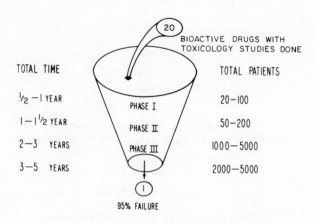

TOTAL TIME

½ – 1 YEAR

1 – 1½ YEAR

2 – 3   YEARS

3 – 5   YEARS

20

BIOACTIVE DRUGS WITH
TOXICOLOGY STUDIES DONE

TOTAL PATIENTS

20 – 100

50 – 200

1000 – 5000

2000 – 5000

PHASE I

PHASE II

PHASE III

1

95% FAILURE

FIG. 1.   The safety evaluation of new drugs.

there could be no human research and no therapeutic progress.   Indeed,
if doing no harm were the main objective of medical practitioners,
they would dare not administer penicillin or digitalis; they would
dare not perform surgery; they would dare not treat any patients.
All medical practice is actually clinical research.   Indeed, every
time a physician treats any patient, he is engaging in a "first-time"
and unique experiment.   If one's primary objective is to do no harm,
he should not only do no research, he should leave the practice of
medicine.   The goal of the clinical practitioner is to help sick
people.   In helping sick people, one constantly accepts the intrinsic risks in light of the greater therapeutic gains.

We have been exposed to several ideas on the purposes of Phase I.
I'd like to present mine from the point of view of an investigator.
Table 1 shows the objectives for Phase-I testing.   In my opinion,
one doesn't ascertain the safety of a drug in Phase I, or for that
matter in Phase II or III.   There are many examples of drugs which
have been marketed in the United States long before serious toxicity
was recognized.   The reason for this is that when the incidence of
a blood dyscrasia is perhaps 1 in 40,000, as with Monase, or 1 in
30,000 to 60,000, as with chloramphenicol, one simply will not or-
dinarily learn this during Phase I, II, or III, when only perhaps

TABLE 1

Phase I Objectives

Tolerance and dose-range in man (usually "normals")

Absorption-excretion $T_{\frac{1}{2}}$

Occasionally a "feel" for efficacy

Occasionally drug metabolism and mechanism of action

Confirm reliability of a new animal or biochemical screen

---

3 to 5,000 patients receive the drug. There are other examples:
Parnate and the tyramine-related hypertensive crises, etc. In my
opinion, Phase-I studies only give one "a feel" for the drug's activity.

Now, to get some of an investigator's specific and practical
problems other than dosage in undertaking Phase I, see Figure 2
depicting the modern harassed clinical investigator. He has pres-
sures and problems from a variety of sources. These include more
sophisticated patients; medical colleagues who don't regard clinical
pharmacology as a mature, or even important, specialty; pharmaceutical and government sponsors who by the nature of their jobs must add
to the problems of the clinical investigator; lawyers who insist
that the principle consideration in human research is protection of

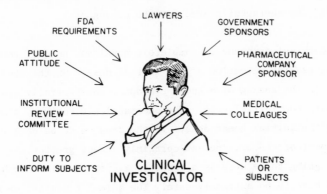

FIG. 2.   Problems of a clinical researcher.

individual freedom and rights (rather than the good of humanity or
therapeutic progress); ever increasing FDA requirements; a public
attitude which is suspicious, at least, toward physicians who "experiment"; institutional review committees which are largely composed
of nonclinical investigators and nonphysicians who presumably are
more capable and interested in protecting a patient's well-being than
the physician-investigator; and finally the duty to inform subjects--
a serious responsibility, but perhaps an impossible one, especially
with experimentation in Phases I and II, when side effects are really
not yet known.

As a clinical investigator who has been active almost 25 years
in human research, I've never yet heard of too large a dose being
used in the initial studies in man. It might have happened, but I am
not aware of it. Far more often, the contrary happens. That is, we
have occasionally ended up giving 30 or more pills to an individual
in a single-dose study because the bioactivity was grossly over-
estimated from pharmacological data.

The initial human dose depends on the following:

1. The nature of the chemical compound
2. The nature of pharmacologic activity
3. The animal toxicology results
4. The availability and reliability of human methodology
5. The therapeutic need for the new agent

If a chemical compound is completely novel and unique, this certainly
influences the selection of the initial dose. On the other hand, if
it is in the analog of a known compound, one generally can better
estimate the initial dose. The pharmacologic activity also influences the initial human dose. If the drug is to be used in the
treatment of cancer, one can certainly accept greater toxicity. If
it is going to be used as a cosmetic agent, on the other hand, it
would have to be extremely safe. The animal toxicity, as has been
emphasized, greatly influences the selection of the initial human

dose.   Did anything unusual occur in the animal toxicity studies?
What are the particular parameters one has to search for in man that
occurred in the animal?

But our major difficulties revolve around the protocol.   (Fig.
3)   I think biostatisticians are being permitted excessive authority
in government and in industry, in designing clinical protocols as
well as in interpreting results.   I think it's often a matter of the
physician's submissiveness because he doesn't understand their language.   They often sit on protocol or other committees, listen quietly to toxicologists, pharmacologists, and clinicians assembling the
pieces of a study, and they're like a poker player quietly holding a
royal flush.   They announce that the study can't be meaningful without four parallel, randomized, stratified groups with 25 subjects
per group.   Subjects must all be within ±10% of ideal body weight,
be males between 21 and 36, be hospitalized and observed 30 days,

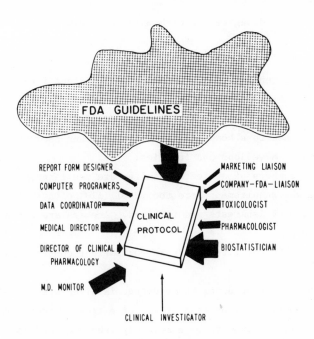

FIG. 3.   The clinical protocol

and have normal SMA-60's. Biostatisticians need to get away from
the biological bias often accumulated from backgrounds involving
data generated by cages of mice and dogs. They need to get the feel
of morning rounds on a hospital ward, together with some apprecia-
tion for sick people; often people with multiple diagnoses, on multiple medications, with anxieties, time problems, family problems,
and economic problems. The biostatistician should be a service to
clinical pharmacologists and not their pristine ruler.

Clinical investigators interact almost exclusively with company
monitors or research associates. We don't usually negotiate protocols with FDA people. Now the industry monitor is, of course, not
a free man either. He doesn't write the protocol all alone. It is
the very sophisticated product of a committee. Each of these individuals brings with him a different set of experiences and biases,
along with a wealth of information. The result is often a 20-page
compendium.

My principle disagreement with many protocols is that they're
getting impractical:

1. They often require "vibrant health," except for one pure
    and excruciating disease.
2. They usually require a large number of young adult males
    confined to a hospital, whereas our young healthy males
    mostly have jobs and families.
3. The numbers of subjects required are too large.
4. Weight requirements are too ideal (±10% of normal).
5. Too many lab tests are required. Anemias are often iatro-
    genic.
6. There is too little concern for patient comfort and conven-
    ience.
7. Too strict an upper range dosage is often stipulated. In
    my opinion, if no side effect or efficacy occurs, the doses
    should continue to be cautiously increased and the study
    continued.

8. They try to answer too many questions with one study. Too
    often a novice monitor attempts to ascertain dosage, effi-
    cacy, safety, and even mechanisms and half-life, from a sin-
    gle study of perhaps only six patients.
9. Often the report forms don't reflect the protocol require-
    ments, i.e., many more unexpected items suddenly appear out
    of the blue on the report forms.

I've tried to recite some of our problems--the investigator's
problems--with the first human dose and with the protocol, but the
major problem in experimental clinical research today is consumerism, i.e., an overemphasis of the rights of the individual in our
society. Too few fight for therapeutic progress. Too few fight
for the rights and greater benefit of mankind. It's not popular to
to talk or publish papers about drug efficacy, but if your paper is
about drug toxicity, JAMA and the New York Times--let alone the
Washington Post--will give you top coverage.

If your "thing" is drug surveillance, you can get millions of
dollars in support from government and foundations. If your "thing"
is trying to do everyday Phase I, II, and III, or to get funds to
train young MD's to learn how to test drug efficacy, very little
money can be found!

Our government spent billions in our moon exploration projects.
I happen to have favored that project, but almost everyone agrees
that putting men into a foreign environment, i.e., space, carries
a real risk (eight died), and the benefits were not universally accepted. Throughout the space explorations, when the astronauts
returned, they were usually instant international heroes; they had
instant promotions and decorations. The president phoned them and
had them to the White House for dinner, and he sent them around the
world as ambassadors of American technology.

To me, putting men into a foreign environment is very similar
to putting, in the form of an experimental pill, a new foreign environment into man. There is a real uncertainty. The benefits

are dubious in early Phase I and the risks are real. But when the
study is completed and perhaps a new therapeutic agent is eventually
confirmed, don't wait for any presidential phone calls or decorations.
If the benefits outweigh the risks of the new drug, the lonely investigator and the company and FDA may sigh with relief that things went
safely and well, but there will be no ticker tape parades for you.
The major difference, in my opinion, is that public sentiment sup-
ports the one program and not the other.

I should remind you that since 95% of the new drugs given to man
fail to show a favorable benefit-to-risk ratio, the vast majority of
the time we clinical investigators live with failure. The risks of
95% of the new drugs outweigh the benefits, so they are abandoned.
Our hope is that we can minimize the danger to the patient. We indeed conduct research at our own peril, too. While we are waiting
for another penicillin or cortisone or cancer cure to come along,
we must aim our efforts at our primary goal, i.e., trying to learn
the truth about new drugs--whether good or bad.

Chapter 4

THE ROLE OF A PRIVATE ORGANIZATION
IN DRUG DISCOVERY AND DEVELOPMENT

Stephen L. DeFelice*

Clinical Resources, Inc.
New York, New York

When I was first trying to prepare this paper, I think the title
was "The Role of a Private Organization in the First Human Dose."
I couldn't get quite excited over that. And I was thumbing through
the transcripts of the Nelson hearings and became depressed. And
then I became disturbed. So I decided to change the paper. I decided to write about the freedom in our culture to be able to study
a compound at all. I háve therefore changed the title to "The Role
of a Private Organization in Drug Discovery and Development."

I'd like to make a hypothesis that's been made before, but to
which no one seems to want to listen or respond. The hypothesis is
that there is a direct correlation between the freedom of drug evaluation and the discovery of drugs. Any system, therefore, which un-
duly hinders human experimentation will result in decreased drug
discovery. To those of you who are excited about preclinical screens,
have a martini some night and think about what these screens tell you.
They don't tell you that much. Think about the fact that many drugs
were discovered in man by serendipity, and continue to be. Think how
critical it is to be able to test a hypothesis in man. Without this

*Present address: Bio-Basics International, New York, New York

privilege there can be no progress. Look at the past decade and
remember that it's extremely difficult to clinically evaluate a drug.
Litigation, guidelines, peer groups, and other hindrances have inex-
orably multiplied. And what have you seen in the past decade? A
decrease in drug discovery. The hypothesis, gentlemen, is justified.
Who's talking about it? When people mention it they are rebuked
with words such as "Auschwitz." And, by the way, the hindrances are
not about to go away. We'll talk about that later. So what's going
on? Why don't we have a good drug-discovery system? Why is it difficult to put a drug into man? What's going to happen? What can we
do about it?

Let's look at the components of the system. First, let's take
a look at the FDA. It always puzzles me why the academic community
looks to FDA to handle the problem of drug discovery. Legislatively
and historically it's not supposed to and hasn't done so. Commis-
sioner Edwards has stated more than once that the responsibility of
the FDA is not drug discovery, but the protection of the public.
One way of doing it is to limit the use of drugs by people. And
they're doing a very good job of that. An inevitable side effect of
this endeavor, however, is to limit the degree of freedom in clinical research. It's a paradox that the organization that has the
most control over clinical investigation and, thereby, on our drug
discovery system, is not concerned with drug discovery.

Let's look at the pharmaceutical industry, the second component
of the system. I think it was Silk of the New York Times who said
that the FDA is always reacting instead of acting. This is also
true of the pharmaceutical industry. The pharmaceutical industry
is constantly reacting to forces outside its control. As a result,
the brainpower of this industry is now tied up in defensive activity
such as product survival. It is not sufficiently involved in the
process of drug discovery. This is particularly pertinent when one
considers that there is more medical brainpower in a local hospital
than in one large pharmaceutical firm. Clinical research is now
cookbookish and controlled by unimaginative guidelines. Though

applied research is necessary, when it becomes a predominant part of the system it is time to be careful. To be sure, these things are difficult to quantify. Yet when you live with them they are easy to understand.

As to the academic community, I still maintain the position that it is not sufficiently aware of the principles of clinical drug development. We have lots of specialists and lots of experts. But the big-picture people, the pragmatists, the great men are rare, simply because it is not a primary function of academics to function as drug discoverers. Then, lastly, we have the National Institute of Health, which is not in the business of discovering drugs either, though it is doing a fine job of funding basic research and training clinical investigators.

So what do we have? We have a system that is discordant and nonproductive, despite the fact that technology, the academic community, and the pharmaceutical industry are better than ever, and despite the fact that the FDA is more sophisticated. It is becoming extremely difficult to clinically evaluate a hypothesis, resulting in a dampening of inspiration. There is nothing that kills inspiration like waiting six or seven years for basic and clinical scientists to see whether the compound can pass the FDA. Should we blame it on the FDA? No. We would be fools to do that. This phenomenon is part of the larger picture. There is something going on in our culture in which all these components are caught. The word that is used to describe this phenomenon is "consumerism." The spirit of consumerism stresses the rights of the individual over those of society—that is, the particular good is more important than the general good. Civilized societies usually tend to move in this direction. Indeed, automobiles may have been made safer by Nader's encounter with General Motors, but his meddling in Dr. Belton's division can only delay drugs that will ameliorate morbidity and delay mortality. It is this failure to recognize the paradoxical effect of consumerism that is having a negative effect on drug discovery.

Will it get worse? Wait until technology improves! The FDA seems to be confident about the application of the risk-to-benefit ratio--a concept I find difficult to apply except in extreme conditions. When technology improves and we see cytoplasmic membranes doing peculiar things and are able to detect mutagenicity at minute dose levels, theoretical risk-benefit will become a more powerful force--a force preventing further evaluation of drugs in man. It's clear. It's on the horizon.

And finally, we have the Congress. And what has the Congress done about drug discovery? Not a thing. It doesn't understand the problem. Yet Congressional action is needed to spur on drug discovery. Clearly a partial decentralization of clinical research away from federal control is needed. In other words, bring research back to the academic community, where the experts are. It makes sense, but those of you with the wisdom of the years behind you realize that it won't happen. In addition, there's no movement to make it happen.

There's only one element left that can move the direction of clinical research in its proper direction--academic medicine. Why not? That's where all the brainpower is. That's where most of the talent is. And yet, how do you stimulate this thing? How do you put it together?

What I think is going to happen is that another mechanism, a fifth component of the system, will develop. Let's call it a private organization, for the sake of argument, a third party removed from the adversary role of these other elements of the drug discovery system. This organization will work with academic medicine. It must be exceptionally competent and objective to survive. Its recommendations must be based on facts and not politics. It should not take years, for example, to assess whether phenothiazines are indicated for the treatment of psychoneurotic anxiety. Yet the politics of science still prevents this resolution. In order to avoid the effect of special interest on decision-making, the client--be it FDA, the pharmaceutical industry, or foundations--will

not interact with the academic peer groups during deliberations.
This organization will be the conduit for objectivity and creativity,
thereby increasing productivity. I think only in that way can one
be objective today. In addition, there is some evidence that this
system is a good one. In our organization the use of the isolated
peer-group approach has, so far, been successful. And finally,
these private organizations must have an international capacity to
clinically evaluate drugs. Those of you who are waiting for the
United States to "open up again" with respect to innovation are not
realists. We must go abroad in order to follow new leads with vigor
and sophistication. So the international approach through academia
must be established and must have credibility.

I suspect by 1975 this is going to be a way of life in the
United States. There will be private organizations dealing with
academia alone. If that doesn't happen, I don't see any solution.
I think things will continue to go downhill. More and more lawyers
will be on Gil McMahon's human research committee. More and more
papers will have to be signed. Lawyers, in a very significant way,
will be controlling clinical research. I think that's going to happen. All information will be placed in files, and when something
goes wrong five or ten years later, the investigator will be held
accountable, despite the absence of fault.

Gentlemen, these facts, coupled with the failure of Congress to
act rationally, leads one to pessimism. To those who still cling
to the belief that the United States should continue to lead the
way in drug discovery and development, I say, "First understand the
problem and then speak from the pulpits."

Chapter 5

OTOTOXICITY: ITS DETECTION AND PREVENTION

Robert E. Brummett

University of Oregon Medical School
Portland, Oregon

This discussion concerns the types of data that can be obtained
from animal studies regarding the nature of the detrimental effects
produced by ototoxic drugs. The significance of these findings will
be interpreted in the light of how this data can be useful in detecting ototoxic effects in man.

A large number of drugs are known to deleteriously affect the
ear. Most of these drugs belong to one of three groups: the aminoglycoside antibiotics, the salicylate analgesics, or the loop-
inhibiting diuretics. In addition, it is important to note that
quinine and pamaquine (1) are reported to be ototoxic as well as
topically applied chloramphenacol (2) and cocaine (3). Thalidamide
is reported to produce teratogenic effects that alter the ear (4).

All of the ototoxic drugs known at the present time exert an
effect on the inner ear. This is not surprising because, with the
exception of teratogenic effects, there are few opportunities for
drugs to alter the middle or outer hair structures, as they only
serve as a sound-conducting system.

Almost without exception, the first observation that any of
these drugs were damaging to the ear came from clinical cases; this
did not have to be. All drugs that are known to be ototoxic in
humans can be shown to be ototoxic in other experimental animals.

This means that the ototoxic capability of any drug could have been determined in animal studies before the drug was used in humans. The only obstacle is that you must first have suspicions that the new drug could be ototoxic. That is to say, that if you have any new drug that is chemically or pharmacologically related to known ototoxic compounds, it must be tested for ototoxicity in experimental animals before it is tried in humans. If information as to the nature of the ototoxic lesion produced by a new drug is available before its human use, it is quite probable that many cases of iatrogenic deafness could be prevented.

All known ototoxic drugs exert a damaging effect on the inner ear. Therefore, it is possible to study the nature of these effects by studying the inner ear. For the present discussion we will limit ourselves to drug effects on the cochlear portion of the inner ear. When the effects of a drug on cochlear electrophysiology are examined, coupled with a histological examination of the cochlea, much information can be gained concerning the cochlear involvement of any ototoxic drug. The two electrophysiological parameters that are most often studied are the ability of the cochlea to generate the alternating current (a.c.) cochlear potential and the gross evoked potential from the VIII nerve (N_1). The a.c. cochlear potential is an electrical analog of the sound that initiated it. That is to say, when a 1000-Hz tone is introduced into the ear, the cochlea generates a 1000-Hz a.c. potential. It is felt, at the present time, that this a.c. potential is generated when the hair cells in the organ of Corti are bent by the vibratory action of the sound entering the cochlea via the stapes footplate (Fig. 1). The gross evoked potential of the VIII nerve is presumably generated in the cochlear portion of the VIII nerve and is the result of the simultaneous firing of large numbers of nerve fibers in response to tone pulses. The N_1 potential is therefore obtained from a structure one step closer to the central nervous system than is the a.c. cochlear potential. Both the a.c. cochlear potential and N_1 can be recorded from an electrode that is placed on the round-window membrane.

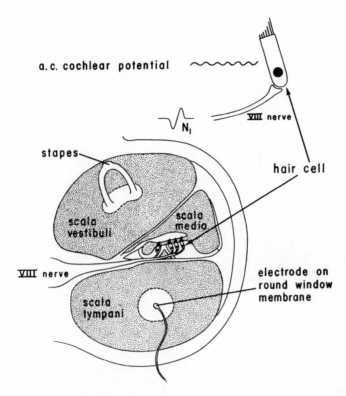

FIG. 1. A schematic drawing of a cross-section of the cochlea showing the relative locations of the stapes (vibratory input into the inner ear) and the round-window membrane (site of electrophysiological recording). The assumed generators for the a.c. cochlear potential and N_1 are also depicted.

Electronic equipment needed to record the a.c. cochlear potential and N_1 is shown in Figure 2.

The effect of the ototoxic aminoglycoside antibiotic, gentamicin, on the cochlea's ability to generate the a.c. cochlear potential is shown in Figure 3 (5). This type of data presentation is often referred to as a sensitivity function. It represents the amount of sound (vertical axis) that is required by the ear involved to generate 1 μV of a.c. cochlear potential at various sound frequencies (horizontal axis). In many ways, this plot can be compared with an audiogram, in that the ability of the cochlea to function at various frequencies is being tested. The range of this 1-μV isopotential

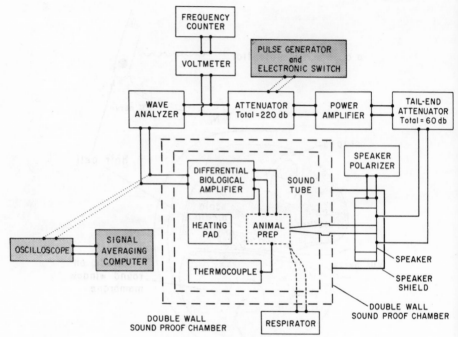

FIG. 2. A block diagram of the equipment required to elicit
and monitor the a.c. cochlear potential and nerve-evoked response
(N_1). For recording the a.c. cochlear potential only the equipment
shown in the open boxes is required; for the recording of N_1 the
equipment shown in the stippled boxes is added.

sensitivity function in four control animals that received the drug
vehicle for 4 weeks is shown in the shaded area. The same type of
data is shown for four individual animals who had received differing
daily doses of gentamicin subcutaneously. It can be seen that the
first effect is the loss of the ability of the cochlea to generate
the a.c. cochlear potential at high frequencies. At the same time,
the cochlea's ability to generate the a.c. cochlear potential is
relatively unaffected at the low frequencies. However, as the daily
dose of drug is increased, or the duration of its administration
extended, the effect progresses so that it eventually involves both
low and high frequencies.

    In addition to the ability to generate very small amounts of
a.c. cochlear potential, there is a large intensity range over which
the cochlea can function. When the intensity of the sound being
introduced into the ear is increased, the cochlea responds by gener-

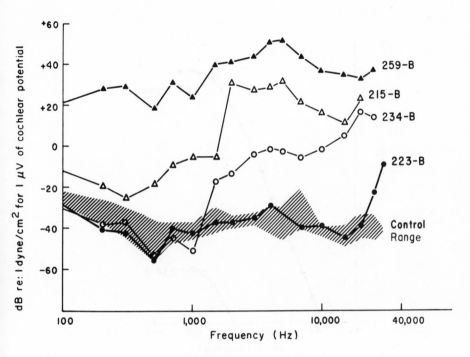

FIG. 3.   The 1-μV isopotential sensitivity function obtained
from four control animals (hatched area) and four individually
labeled animals who had received large doses of gentamicin.

ating increased amounts of a.c. cochlear potential. This process
increases until the sound stimulus becomes so intense that it
interferes with cochlear function. When this occurs, further increases in sound intensity will decrease the amount of a.c. cochlear
potential obtained. Figure 4 is an example of this kind of intensity function. It portrays the data obtained at 10 kHz from one of
the gentamicin-treated animals whose 1-μV sensitivity function is
shown in Figure 3. For comparison, the data obtained from a single
control animal is also depicted. In the case of the drug-treated
animal, only 3.4 μV could be produced, while the vehicle treated
animal was able to generate 280 μV. For further comparisons, Table
1 lists the maximum amount of a.c. cochlear potential obtained at
10 kHz and 1 kHz from all of the animals presented in Figure 3.

     A drug-induced decrease in the ability of the cochlea to gener-
ate the a.c. cochlear potential is often accompanied by the

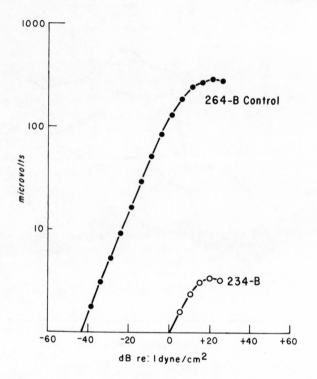

FIG. 4.   The intensity function of the a.c. cochlear potential
obtained at 10 kHz from a single control animal (264-B) and a
single gentamicin treated animal (234-B).

TABLE 1

Maximum A.C. Cochlear Potential in Gentamicin-treated Animals

Animal No.	Daily Dose (mg/kg)	Duration (weeks)	Max. a.c. cochlear potential (µV)	
			1,000 Hz.	10,000 Hz.
234-B	100	2	18	3.4
223-B	50	4	960	170
215-B	100	4	12.5	1.1
259-B	150	4	29	2.1
Control		4	1119	304

destruction of cochlear hair cells. In the data presented here, the
condition of the hair cells was determined by the surface preparation
technique of Engstrom et al. (6). In this case, the cochlea was
fixed with 1% osmium tetroxide. After fixation and serial dehydration to 70% ethanol, the cochlea was dissected using microdissection
tools. Segments of the basilar membrane from all turns of the cochlea were mounted in glycerin and the hair cells were visualized with
a phase-contrast microscope. By focusing down on the hair cells it
can easily be determined when cells are missing from the organ of
Corti. Figure 5 shows a photomicrograph of the hair cells as viewed
by this technique. Missing-hair-cell data is presented as a recon-
struction of the cochlea as shown in Figure 6. The areas in the
cochlea from which the hair cells are missing determine the effect
on cochlear function. The basal turn of the cochlea is involved in
the transduction of high frequency sound and the apical turn is involved with low frequencies. In the animal shown, the basal turn
is almost totally destroyed while the apical turns are unaffected.
The correlation between the hair cell damage in the animal and the
sensitivity function of the a.c. cochlear potential can be seen by
referring back to Figure 3.

A very important point must be made about the data concerning
the electrophysiology of the cochlea. It does not represent
"hearing." In order for an animal to hear, the entire auditory system must be involved. Data on the electrophysiology of the cochlea
only tells us that the cochlea is able to transduce acoustical sig-
nals into its analogous a.c. cochlear potential. Because this is
one of the early steps involved in hearing, when it is interferred
with, hearing is also interferred with.

The data presented thus far was obtained after the administration of a rather large dose of an aminoglycoside for a considerably
long time period. After drug administration had been terminated,
a period of about 2 weeks was allowed to lapse for the drug damage
to stabilize. The resultant data represent the end result of the
drug insult to the ear but do not reveal the time course over which

A
3
2
1
OHC
T
IHC
B
OHC
T
IHC

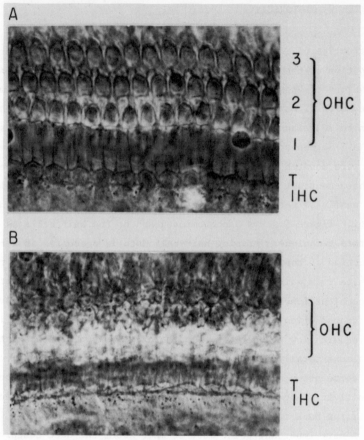

FIG. 5. Surface preparations of the hair cells of the guinea pig cochlea. (A) Obtained from a guinea pig who had received a single subcutaneous dose of 400 mg/kg of kanamycin 30 days prior to sacrifice; the cochlea reveals no hair cell damage. (B) Obtained from a guinea pig who had received a single 400 mg/kg subcutaneous dose of kanamycin followed in 2 hours by a single 100 mg/kg intravenous dose of furosemide 30 days prior to sacrifice; the cochlea reveals total hair-cell destruction.

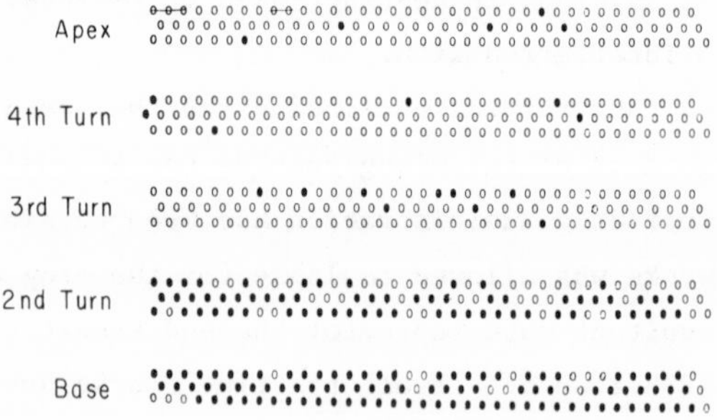

Apex
4th Turn
3rd Turn
2nd Turn
Base

FIG. 6. A schematic representation of the outer hair cells from the indicated cochlear segments. A darkened spot represents a missing hair cell. This is guinea pig 234-B.

the damage occurs.   Data showing the onset of the ototoxic lesion
are found in Figure 7.   In addition, these data more closely approxi-
mate studies involving hearing.   When rather intense tone pulses are
presented to rodents, they respond with a twitch of the pinna.   This
pinna response to a sound stimulus is known as the Preyer pinna reflex.   Whether this represents "hearing" is a moot point; however,
it does represent a physiological reaction in response to sound.
In Figure 7, the stippled area represents the control range of the
sound intensity required to elicit a threshold Preyer pinna reflex
in a single animal (7).   This data was obtained daily over a 3-day
period.   The animal was then given a 400 mg/kg subcutaneous injection of kanamycin every 6 hours until a total of five such doses
had been given.   After this time period no more drug was administered.
Two hours after the last dose, the threshold curve labeled Day 1 was
obtained.   It can be seen that no effect is evident on the Preyer
pinna-reflex threshold.   The threshold curve labeled Day 3 was

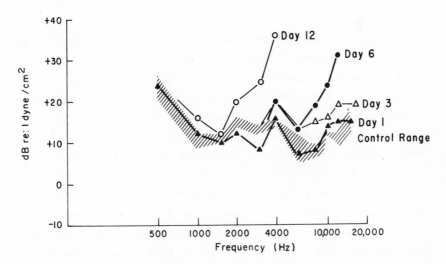

FIG. 7.   Preyer pinna reflex threshold data for a single guinea
pig.   The hatched area represents the range of the threshold obtained daily for 3 days prior to the administration of 400 mg/kg of
kanamycin subcutaneously every 6 hours for a total of five doses.
Day 1 data was obtained 2 hours after the last dose.

obtained 2 days later and shows a slight elevation of the threshold
at high frequencies. This effect progressed until it had stabilized
by the twelfth day. As was seen with the electrophysiology data,
the high frequencies are the first to be affected and the damage progresses to involve lower and lower frequencies.

The concentration of kanamycin in the perilymph of guinea pigs
subjected to the same dose schedule is about 60 γ/ml 4 hours after
the first dose and about 70 γ/ml 4 hours after the last dose. The
concentration of kanamycin in the perilymph decreases with a half-
time of about 15 hours. This means that for about 24 hours the perilymph contains a high and rather constant amount of kanamycin. It
is obvious that the delayed onset of the ototoxic lesion after the
administration of kanamycin is not just a function of the time required to accumulate sufficient drug in the inner ear. It takes
about 3 days before ototoxic effect is manifest. This data would
also suggest that the ototoxic damage can continue for at least a
short period of time, even though the administration of kanamycin
has stopped.

Interactions between drugs known to be ototoxic can also be determined in experimental animals. It has been postulated that much
of the permanent deafness that has been reported following the intravenous injection of ethacrynic acid occurs in those patients who are
simultaneously receiving an aminoglycoside antibiotic (8, 9). To
see if this postulated interaction could be demonstrated in experimental animals, the following experiment was performed (10):

Groups of guinea pigs were anesthetized and prepared for recording the a.c. cochlear potential. They were then given a single 400
mg/kg dose of kanamycin.[*] A 2-hour time period was allowed to
elapse so that the kanamycin would be in the perilymph of the inner
ear. At this time, sufficient sound at 1000 Hz was delivered to
the ear to produce 150 μV of a.c. cochlear potential. This amount

---

[*]We have been unable to ever detect any cochlear damage from a single dose of kanamycin even when doses as high as 800 mg/kg are
given subcutaneously. (Fig. 5)

of sound is not damaging to the ear.   After the sound had been turned
on, a single 40 mg/kg dose of ethacrynic acid was given intravenously.
The end of this 1-minute intravenous-injection period is considered
to be zero time on the horizontal axis of Figure 8.   The a.c. cochlear potential that the cochlea generated to this constant 1000-Hz
tone was then continuously monitored over a 3- to 4-hour period.

It can be seen from Figure 8 that kanamycin followed by an intravenous dose of saline did not alter the cochlea's ability to generate
the a.c. cochlear potential.   It can also be noted that a single
intravenous dose of ethacrynic acid given 2 hours after a subcutaneous dose of saline produces only a temporary effect.   That is,
there was an initial decrease in the a.c. cochlear potential but it

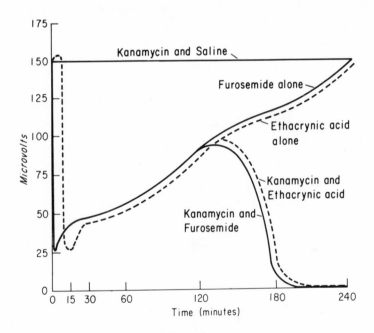

FIG. 8.   Schematic representation of the interaction effect
between the loop-inhibiting diuretics and kanamycin on the ability
of the cochlea to generate the a.c. cochlear potential at 1 kHz.
The zero time is 2 hours after the subcutaneous injection of 400
mg/kg of kanamycin and immediately after the intravenous injection
of 40 mg/kg ethacrynic acid (or 100 mg/kg of furosemide).

returned towards normal over a 3- to 4-hour period. On the other
hand, when ethacrynic acid was given after kanamycin, an initial
drop of the cochlear output was seen. This effect is indistinguish-
able from the drop produced by ethacrynic acid alone for about 2
hours. At this time, the a.c. cochlear potential falls rapidly to
zero. This is a permanent effect, in that when animals so exposed
are examined 30 days after drug exposure, practically no hair cells
are found in the cochlea (Fig. 5). Furosemide produces a very similar response that can also be seen in Figure 8. However, in the
case of furosemide, a higher dose is required to produce the same
effect (11). This may explain the lack of clinical reports impli-
cating furosemide and kanamycin interactions.

So far we have only mentioned drug insults to the ear that result in permanent cochlear dysfunction. The salicylate drugs have
long been known to produce temporary deafness. Figure 9 shows the
electrophysiological parameters of cochlear function as altered by
a rather large dose of sodium salicylate (12). In this case, groups
of four guinea pigs, at various time intervals after a single 500
mg/kg subcutaneous dose of sodium salicylate, were studied along

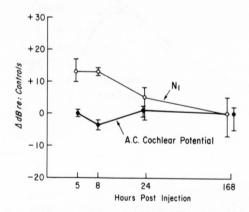

FIG. 9.   Changes in the ability of the guinea pig cochlea to
generate both the a.c. cochlear potential and N_1 at various time
intervals after a single 500 mg/kg subcutaneous dose of sodium
salicylate. There were four drug-treated and two control animals
at each point. The vertical bars represent the range of the data.

with a similar group of two guinea pigs who received an equivalent
volume of saline. All measurements were conducted in a double-blind
manner.

In Figure 9, the zero on the vertical axis represents the mean
sound intensity required to produce 1 µV of a.c. cochlear potential
or 50 µV of N_1 in the control animals. N_1, as you recall, is the
summed nerve-evoked potential. It can be seen from the figure that
very little change occurred in the ability to generate the a.c.
cochlear potential. If anything, it took slightly less sound to
generate this potential 8 hours after the drug. In the case of N_1,
however, the animals required 12 dB more sound to generate 50 µV of
N_1, 5 and 8 hours after the dose of sodium salicylate. At this time
blood salicylate was approximately 40 mg%. At the end of 168 hours,
the ability of the cochlea to generate the a.c. cochlear potential
and N_1 was back to that of the control animals. This indicates a
temporary effect on the cochlea.

Patients who are taking doses of salicylate large enough to produce a temporary hearing loss often report tinnitus. Similarly,
patients exposed to other noxious insults to the ear, such as acous-
tic trauma, aminoglycoside antibiotics, or the loop-inhibiting diuretics, complain of tinnitus. Because tinnitus seems to be often
associated with damage to the ear, it would be very nice to be able
to detect electrophysiological manifestations of tinnitus in experimental animals. At the present time, we have been unable to do this.
Unfortunately, we do not even know if animals other than man can
experience tinnitus. A detection of an auditory hallucination such
as tinnitus in an experimental animal is a difficult feat. When or
if tinnitus can be detected in experimental animals, electrophysiological correlates may then be established and studied as an indicator of toxicity to the cochlea.

If one takes the data from Figure 3 and converts it to the form
seen in human audiograms, one obtains the data depicted in Figure
10. In this case the dB notations below the zero indicate that it
took that much more sound to produce 1 µV of a.c. cochlear potential

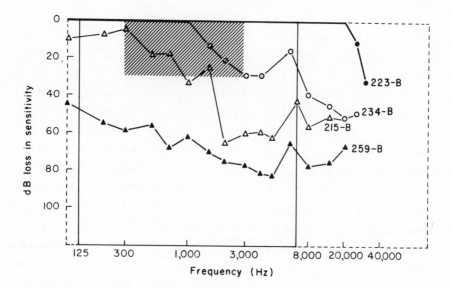

FIG. 10. The 1-µV isopotential sensitivity functions of the gentamicin-treated animals shown in Figure 3. The data is presented as an audiogram. The zero represents the sound intensity required to produce 1 µV of a.c. cochlear potential at each indicated frequency for the worst control animal. The dB below the zero line represents increasing amounts of sound required to produce the 1 µV of a.c. cochlear potential. 125 Hz to 8,000 Hz represents the frequency range of conventional audiometers. The hatched area represents the range of sound intensity and frequency that are required for normal communication. When auditory thresholds are below the hatched area, normal verbal communication is impaired.

than it did in the worst case among the control animals. This would be called dB hearing loss on human audiograms. Several points are significant here and deserve mention. The first is that the conventional audiometer only measures hearing thresholds up to 8 kHz while the human ear can hear frequencies as high as 20 kHz. Animal 223-B exhibited considerable loss in ability to generate the a.c. cochlear potential at frequencies which would not be detected by an available audiometer.

Equally significant is the fact that patients do not usually complain of hearing deficits until they show considerable hearing losses in the speech frequencies. The speech frequencies are

usually considered to be between 300 and 3000 Hz. Only when the
audiological thresholds drop below 30 dB in this range do patients
complain of hearing losses. This means that, if the nature of the
deficit is permanent, the patient can detect hearing losses himself
only when he has a permanent communication problem.

For these reasons, it becomes imperative to at least do an
audiometric evaluation of hearing thresholds when studying any new
drug suspected of producing hearing losses. It would be preferable
to study the frequencies up to the highest that any given patient
is capable of hearing. Only in this way can the earliest manifestations of ototoxicity be detected. If threshold changes were to
be detected when they had only occurred at the very high frequencies,
the drug administration could be stopped or the dosage lowered so as
to prevent the hearing losses from becoming so great as to include
the frequencies involved in communication.

It seems to me that any new drug that is related to any known
ototoxic drug should be evaluated in animals for ototoxicity before
it is tried in man. The correlation in toxicity studies concerning
the ear is very good between man and experimental animals. I also
feel that any drug that is intended to be used in the ear, including
the external or middle ear, should be studied in animals to determine if the preparations are damaging the cochlea. Only by knowing
what to expect can one prevent iatrogenic hearing dysfunction by
drugs.

REFERENCES

1. D. Hennebert and C. Fernandez, Arch. Otolaryngol., 70:321 (1959).

2. G. O. Proud, H. Mittelman, and G. D. Seiden, Arch. Otolaryngol.,
    87:580 (1968).

3. M. Comeau, R. E. Brummett, and J. Vernon, Arch. Otolaryngol.,
    98:114 (1973).

4. G. E. Shambaugh, Jr., "Surgery of the Ear," 2nd ed., W. B.
    Saunders Co., Philadelphia, 1967, p. 408.

5. R. E. Brummett, D. Himes, B. Saine, and J. Vernon, Arch.

Otolaryngol., <u>96</u>:505 (1972).

6. H. Engström, H. W. Ades, and A. Andersson, "Structural pattern of the organ of Corti," Almquist and Wiksell, Stockholm, 1966.

7. P. Herman, D. Anderson, and R. E. Brummett, Manuscript in preparation.

8. A. H. Johnson and C. H. Hamilton, <u>S. Med. J.</u>, <u>63</u>:511 (1970).

9. W. D. Meriwether, R. J. Mangi, and A. A. Serpick, <u>J. Amer. Med. Ass.</u>, <u>216</u>:795 (1971).

10. B. A. West, R. E. Brummett, D. Himes, <u>Arch. Otolaryngol.</u>, <u>98</u>:32 (1973).

11. J. Traynor, R. E. Brummett, and D. Himes, <u>Acta Otolaryngologica</u>, accepted for publication.

12. C. Mitchell, R. E. Brummett, D. Himes, and J. Vernon, <u>Arch. Otolaryngol.</u>, <u>98</u>:297 (1973).

Chapter 6

IS CARCINOGENESIS A PROBLEM?

Jack L. Radomski

Department of Pharmacology
University of Miami School of Medicine

There are several answers to the question, Is carcinogenesis a problem? depending on the interpretation given. If we mean, Do the government and the pharmaceutical companies have a problem with the possible carcinogenic action of drugs? the answer is, unquestionably, You'd better believe it! If by the question we mean, Is carcinogenesis from the ingestion and the administration of drugs a problem? the answer is a great deal more complicated.

Very little is really known about the carcinogenic action of drugs. One reason is that most of our knowledge of chemical carcinogenesis comes from animal experiments, but most drugs, even those where chronic administration to people is likely, have not been studied by lifetime testing in experimental animals. For example, I was amazed a couple of years ago to review the carcinogenic literature on aspirin. There has not been a single chronic feeding experiment conducted with this substance. The maximum exposure has been one year, which is totally inadequate for carcinogenic purposes.

A second reason, I think, is that most drugs are only given to specific people for specific reasons, and are administered by a physician. Therefore, there is a general feeling that if anything goes wrong it will be picked up. This is not the case with food additives, for example, which enter the diet of the entire country.

Were a carcinogenic effect to occur following an additive's release
by the government and its ingestion by people of this country, there
would be very little likelihood of picking it up epidemiologically.
If not tested before released, we would never find out whether an
additive has any subtly deleterious effects.

A third reason why little is known about the carcinogenic action
of drugs is that there is at least a subconscious reluctance on the
part of industry and government alike, I think, to pay attention to
what promises to be a costly and troublesome problem for both. I'm
afraid, however, that at the present moment the can of worms has
been opened and reality must be faced.

Interest in this area has been stimulated by the discovery of
the involvement of nitrogen-containing compounds in carcinogenesis.
I had the occasion to go through Goodman and Gilman (1), drug by
drug and structure by structure, and it's amazing how many drugs
contain nitrogen and are, by one description or another, amines.
They make up close to 90% of all drugs. Apparently, by and large,
if you don't have nitrogen in the structure you don't have a bio-
logically-active compound.

The first group of compounds to be implicated were the nitrosamines. Nitrosamines are among the most potent chemical carcinogens
known to man. They are carcinogenic to the liver, esophagus, G.I.
tract, skin, and almost any tissue they come into contact with. As
long as the nitrosamines were considered an industrial problem, it
seemed as though we only had to be concerned about possible occupa-
tional exposure to these compounds. Then it was discovered that
secondary amines could react with nitrite in an acid medium with
the resultant production of nitrosamines (2). Considering that
nitrites are a fairly common food additive, particularly as a pre-
servative in hot dogs and other sausages, and the secondary amines
are present in fish and other foods, this is a very disquieting
observation. It raised the spectre of possible production within
the stomach and G.I. tract of nitrosamines from a combination of
food components.

The observation was then extended to tertiary amines which can also react with nitrite under mildly acidic conditions to produce nitrosamines. Dr. W. Lijinski carried out in vitro incubation studies at acid pH's with five tertiary-amine drugs and sodium nitrite at 37°C (3). With oxytetracycline, after 4 hours there is a 65% conversion of the oxytetracycline to dimethylnitrosamine. Aminopyrene is 73% converted to dimethylnitrosamine; tolazamide is 28% converted; and disulfiram 6.2% converted. These experiments emphasize the possibility that any drug which is a secondary or tertiary amine may react in the body with nitrite ions ingested in meat and sausages. In addition, it is well known that there are bacteria present in the G.I. tract (e.g. E. coli) which can reduce nitrate to nitrite. (Nitrates are present, sometimes in considerable concentrations, in drinking water.)

The second area of involvement of nitrogen compounds in carcinogenesis is N-oxidation. By N-oxidation we mean the formation of the N-hydroxy, the nitroso, or the N-oxide metabolite of a nitrogen-containing compound. Research in this area began in the Millers' laboratory at McArdle in 1959 with their discovery of N-oxidation (4) and their demonstration that N-hydroxy-2-acetylaminofluorene is the active carcinogenic metabolite of 2-acetylaminofluorene (5). In addition to 2-acetylaminofluorene there are a number of aromatic amines which are N-oxidized and which produce cancer in both man and dog. These are 2-naphthylamine, 4-aminobiphenyl, and benzidene. The N-oxidation of these amines produces N-hydroxy compounds, which may be further oxidized to nitroso compounds--both of these are carcinogenic. These compounds are not nitrosamines, incidentally, but nitroso aromatic compounds which, although perhaps not as well studied nor as potent as nitrosamines, are carcinogenic none the less. Another possibility, demonstrated in our laboratory, is that nitro compounds may be reduced to nitroso and N-hydroxy compounds (6). There are a number of important nitro compounds in medicine such as nitrofurantoin and chloramphenicol.

We were able to show that the N-hydroxy and nitroso compounds of

aromatic amines are the active carcinogens in the induction of bladder cancer, but were concerned by the fact that these compounds are
very unstable and very water soluble. It was known that they were
formed by the liver microsomes, but we could not imagine (1) why
these compounds didn't produce tumors in any tissue except the bladder, and (2) how such stable and water soluble compounds could be
transported from the liver to the bladder to produce their carcinogenic action.

Recent work in our laboratory has demonstrated that this occurs
by the formation of the N-hydroxy compound in the liver, where it
is also conjugated with glucuronic acid (7). We have obtained
strong evidence of the existence of this glucuronic acid conjugate.
This compound is itself inactive. It circulates in the blood but
does not produce tumors in other tissues. It is filtered by the
kidney, enters the urine and is hydrolyzed in the bladder in the
presence of acid and β-glucuronidase to yield the active carcinogens, the N-hydroxy and nitroso compounds.

It was believed at first that N-hydroxylation was a limited phenomenon. However, it is now recognized that N-oxidation is common
with amine drugs. There are a number of different kinds of compounds
which could be N-oxidized. In most cases N-hydroxy compounds are
formed, but sometimes the N-oxide is formed. N-oxides may also be
carcinogenic. Several compounds such as chlorpromazine and sulfa-
nilamide have been demonstrated to be excreted in the urine as N-
oxidized metabolites.

What we have been talking about up to the present time has been
possibilities and potentialities. Lijinsky's work was carried out
with rather high concentrations of nitrites, and it isn't known
whether these observations would apply to the low concentrations of
nitrites that are developed in the stomach or intestine following
the ingestion of sausages and hot dogs. In addition, many of the
drugs which may theoretically produce N-hydroxy metabolites may not
actually do so, since sometimes these compounds are difficult to
form.

To return to the question, then--is carcinogenesis really a problem? Are people developing cancer because of drugs currently being prescribed or sold over the counter? The answer to this is probably, Yes. F.J.C. Rowe, a distinguished British experimenter in chemical carcinogenesis, has compiled a list of relatively high-risk carcinogenic compounds. He contends that it is naive to talk of chemicals as carcinogenic or noncarcinogenic and that they should be talked of in terms of relative risk of carcinogenesis. The list was compiled on the basis of an established correlation between animal tests and clinical and epidemiological investigations in humans. Alkylating agents, used as immunosuppressives and in the therapy of cancer, are also capable of producing cancer. Urethane, which used to be used as a necrotizing agent in the treatment of hemorrhoids, is a carcinogenic compound. Isonicotinic acid hydrazide probably has some risk associated with it. There is no doubt of the carcinogenic action of coal tar, estrogens, and diethylstilbestrol. A combination of I^{131} and goitrogens can cause cancer of the thyroid. Phenacetin in large doses for long periods of time causes renal carcinoma and carcinoma of the bladder (9).

So I think we have to say that people are developing cancer from drugs currently in use. Probably in most instances the risk involved is justified by the therapeutic effects of the drug. But this still doesn't get to the heart of the problem. I think the heart of the problem is a slightly different question: Are drugs currently in use responsible for any significant portion of the cancer problem? And the answer to this is--God only knows! Or worse yet--God only knows how to find out!

What really significant approaches can be made to gather information about the problem?

First, I think it is important to concentrate our efforts in areas where cancer is a large or increasing problem. For example, if a chemical is found which is carcinogenic to the liver in animal studies, it is not too important, since the incidence of liver carcinoma is this country is low and probably decreasing. Stomach carcinogens also would not warrant too much concern. On the other hand, colon cancer and bladder cancer are serious and increasing problems.

Also, resources for research into drug carcinogenesis should be concentrated in areas where there is a good chance that the particular cancer may be drug induced. Bladder cancer, for example, is almost certainly caused by some chemical in the urine. However, it remains an unanswered question whether colon cancer is caused by an orally ingested food additive, drug, virus, or something else. Further research into the causes of specific cancers is needed.

Epidemiological studies ought to be greatly expanded. A great deal can be done. There is thought now being given to computerized registries of prescriptions and attempts to follow up patients to see what eventually happens to them. On a less grandiose scale, I think something simpler can be done. Take a detailed history of patients who have developed certain types of cancer. Ask them about their history, what kinds of chronic diseases they had, and what drugs they took in the past. Amazingly enough, very little of this has been done.

More animal testing is needed. Of course, there should also be an attempt to establish correlations with human cancer. In my field, aromatic amines in carcinogenesis, we have such a correlation. The trouble is, if you observe the carcinogenicity of a compound in an animal, then you can't test it in people. With aromatic amines, it developed the other way around, that is, the observation was made in humans and then it was found that the dog developed the same kind of tumors from the same compound.

I think more metabolic studies need to be done. Metabolic studies usually have the virtue of being possible to carry out in humans because you only have to give a single small dose and analyze the urine. Working the three things together, epidemiological observation, animal tests, and metabolic studies, one can get, I'm sure, a believable picture as to the real carcinogenic action of drugs as it pertains to people—not mice or rats.

REFERENCES

1. L. S. Goodman and A. Gilman, "The Pharmacological Basis of Ther-
    apeutics," Macmillan, New York, 1970.

2. N. P. Sen, D. C. Smith, and L. Schwinghamer, Fd. Cosmet. Toxicol.,
    7:301 (1969).

3. W. Lijinsky, E. Conrad, and R. Van de Bogart, Nature (Lond.),
    239:165 (1972).

4. J. W. Cramer, J. A. Miller, and E. C. Miller, J. Biol. Chem.,
    235:885 (1960).

5. E. C. Miller, J. A. Miller, and H. A. Hartmann, Cancer Res., 21:
    815 (1961).

6. J. L. Radomski, G. M. Conzelman, Jr., A. A. Rey, and E. Brill,
    J. Nat. Cancer Inst., 50:989 (1973).

7. J. L. Radomski, A. A. Rey, and E. Brill, Cancer Res., 33:1284
    (1973).

8. H. Uehleke, "Biological Oxidation of Nitrogen in Organic Mole-
    cules," Taylor and Frances, London, 1972, p. 15.

9. F. J. C. Roe, Clin. Pharmacol. Therap., 7:77 (1966).

Chapter 7

PREDICTION OF EARLY DRUG
TOXICITY: THE IMPOSSIBLE DREAM

John B. Miale

Department of Pathology
University of Miami School of Medicine
and
Jackson Memorial Hospital
Miami, Florida

My interest in the prediction of early drug toxicity arises from
my involvement in laboratory medicine and, specifically, from two
problem areas that I have been facing for many years. The first is
our involvement in the protocols for laboratory studies that are
performed as part of various drug-toxicity studies and drug-investi-
gation programs. The second, of closer interest to me, is the similarity of the question of detection of early drug toxicity to that
of the detection of early disease. The two problems are closely
related, for it has always seemed to me that if one cannot detect
early disease, then one cannot detect early drug toxicity; likewise,
if one cannot detect early drug toxicity, one cannot detect early
disease.

There is much evidence that, in spite of current vogue, we have
so far failed to come up with the means for detecting early disease
in a strict sense. Perhaps I have overstated the problem in the
title of my talk in saying that this is an impossible dream, but I
will give you some of the reasons for my evaluation of the present
state of the art.

Regarding the many ways that drugs can be toxic, today's presentation is directed to those adverse reactions that are detectable by clinical laboratory investigations because a biochemical lesion or biochemical abnormality is produced that is measurable by the usual laboratory tests. We must also assume that what we are aiming toward is the detection of early drug toxicity at a stage preceding advanced or irreversible cell damage. With regard to the analogy to early disease this is, of course, also our goal.

My thesis is that if it is not impossible, it is at least presently very difficult to predict early toxicity and to detect early disease. There are shortcomings in methodology and instrumentation, both from the standpoint of accuracy, that is, a closeness to the true value, and with regard to the precision, that is, reproducibility, of certain determinations. This, perhaps, is a problem that can be solved eventually. But perhaps of even greater importance, at least in my experience, are the very real, and sometimes unappreciated problems in statistics and logic--in the decision of whether a person is normal or abnormal, or whether a test is normal or abnormal. I need not point out that the problem is not in obtaining data (anybody can obtain data), but in determining the significance of data, from both the standpoint of its quality, (based on such factors as accuracy, precision, quality control methods) and its significance to the patient under study.

We can use as a model the currently popular concept of the multichannel chemical screen, of which the Technicon SMA/12 is a good example. This determines 12 chemical constituents in serum and records results automatically on a special chart paper that also gives, for each constituent, a range of "normal." As usually interpreted, if the recorder line for a given determination falls within the crosshatched normal area the value is considered "normal"; if it falls outside of the normal area the value is considered "abnormal."

In spite of current popularity, there are significant limitations to the value of this approach. Sadly, some of these limitations are not generally appreciated.

One of these relates to the significance of the so-called normal range for each biochemical value. For example, the preprinted chart gives the normal range for serum uric acid as 2.5 to 8.0 mg/dl of serum. We know, however, that uric acid concentration in serum is significantly influenced by the age, sex, and ethnic group of the patient. If each variable is taken into account there is a different "normal" range depending on age, sex, and ethnic group. If these are not taken into consideration we are presented with a composite normal range of limited significance. Inevitably, the range is very broad and the likelihood of critical detection of early abnormality is small.

Furthermore, the definition of normality is nothing more than the statistical distribution of values in a group of supposedly asymptomatic and normal individuals. This brings me to the second shortcoming of this particular approach. That is, if we define normality on the basis of the 95% normal range, then in a system of n multiple independent analyses, the probability of all the determinations being normal in a so-called normal individual is 0.95^n. In other words, in screening with 12 independent analyses, as in our example, we should expect that roughly half (0.95^{12}) of the patients will have at least one abnormality, as defined by these ranges, which may or may not be a true abnormality. This is a statistical fact which should not be ignored; yet we find that several ways are used to get around this rather disturbing problem. One way is to decide that we will not interpret the data too closely--we'll only interpret markedly abnormal results as being "clinically significant." Of course, this may be a nice way out for the clinician who is studying obvious disease, but does not do anything to detect occult disease, or in our situation, early drug toxicity. Nevertheless, this type of study is commonly a part of every protocol involving the possible toxic reactions to drugs, and I always wonder what is done with the information that is obtained. It seems to me that usually the report is impressively replete with data like this, whether it means anything or not, and that most of the time it's simply ignored.

I would like to point out one other thing. Within a certain group of so-called normals showing a broad baseline, there could be, in the course of drug administration, a marked change for a given patient (for example, from a serum uric-acid level at approximately 3 to a uric-acid level of approximately 7) that would be highly significant; yet both values would fall within the so-called normal baseline. I'll come back to this again.

We have then the statistical problem in multiple independent analyses, and if we do $\underline{n}$ analyses, the probability that all of these will be within the normal range, defined as the 95% range, would be 0.95^n. As a corollary to this, if one adds more tests to the system, more independent analyses, then the probability of patients showing no abnormalities becomes smaller and smaller. The more complex and more complicated the protocol with regard to multiple analyses, the fewer and fewer patients will turn out to be normal, even though they are normal as far as can be determined clinically. This holds true for the classic 95% range of normality. A similar calculation will show that if one takes three standard deviations as the normal range (97.5%), one gains relatively little, because 0.975^{12} is not much different than 0.95^{12}.

Also, if in addition to this problem of definition of normality, one broadens the base of normal because of less than ideal methodology and instrumentation, then the base becomes broader and broader, and the definition of normality becomes fuzzier in every case.

One study done in my laboratory (1) provides support for my remarks. On 479 patients admitted to our hospital, we performed a multichannel screening which consisted of 17 independent analyses. Of these, 403 had one or more abnormalities, defined as a value falling outside the 95% normal range, and only 76 showed no abnormality. In the group of 403 patients showing one or more abnormality, the abnormality in 356 was either a feature of the patient's disease or it was thought not to be significant, since in about 80% the abnormal value fell within a range of greater than 2 S.D., but smaller than 3 S.D. In the other 20%, the abnormality could be related to the patient's illness. In the remaining 73 patients, significant disease was found in only 28, while in 45 it was felt that no disease was present. The further investigations required to make these decisions are costly and time-consuming, particularly in the nondisease group.

The pertinence of this to the question of detecting early drug toxicity is obvious. One need only substitute "toxicity" and "non-toxicity" for "disease" and "nondisease." Granted that my example deals with a special population, the same type of study has been performed on populations of supposedly normal individuals (2-6); the same reservations have been expressed and the same shortcomings have been pointed out.

On the positive side, there is no doubt that we can do more to improve the detection of early disease and early toxicity. The ideal situation would be a methodology which would yield a bimodal distribution of values; one mode for the normal population and one for the abnormal, with little or no overlap. Interestingly, there are some laboratory data that give this type of distribution, such as those for partial thromboplastin coagulation time. What we usually find, however, is an overlap between high normal values and low abnormal values, and this creates problems of interpretation. In spite of the graphic attractiveness of charts with values expressed in milligram, microgram, or nanogram units, one is still faced with the question of whether these results are significant from the standpoint of detecting early drug toxicity.

We can achieve greater precision if we realize its importance and demand that instrumentation accomplish it. The problem with instrumentation, as far as the clinical laboratory is concerned, is that the manufacturer presents the consumer with an instrument which will or will not do certain things, but is not necessarily designed to serve the purpose of the investigator. The precision of the instrument is not specified by the consumer but by the manufacturer. When I have pointed this out, I have become very unpopular with the manufacturers. It is nevertheless true that we know what we must do, but have not yet been provided with the means.

The second thing that should be accomplished is a better definition of normality. This is one of the great problems in the interpretation of laboratory data, and it is a time-consuming and expen-
sive problem. Strangely enough, when a pharmaceutical company or
some other group is interested in determining toxicity, they want to
assume that we already know what normal values are for the studies
in the protocol. In fact, in many instances we do not know them and,
therefore, the data become less than meaningful. If one is studying
the effects of drugs on young women of child-bearing age, it must be
kept in mind that this group has a totally different set of normal
values than children or geriatric patients or any other group that
one might want to choose.

The third point that I would like to make is that not enough
attention is paid to the follow-up of individual patients. In a
drug protocol, usually a single baseline determination is made of
whatever group of tests are chosen, after which one goes into the
experimental period. I believe that this is not the way to do it.
I think that every subject included in the protocol should at least
have as extensive a baseline study as an experimental period. This
adds to the cost of things, but it is one way by which we can get
meaningful data for each individual patient--the establishment of a
baseline for that patient, which may be quite different from that
for another, and the determination of whether there is a significant
shift in baseline values and whether they fall within the abnormal
range.

In summary, I have pointed out some problems in detecting early
drug toxicity. Since we are not concerned here with alterations so
severe as to be evident clinically, or which produce irrefutably
abnormal biochemical abnormalities, I have emphasized the problem
of interpreting data that lie in the overlapping zone between normality and abnormality. I have also outlined measures that would
yield more accurate and precise data, which would in turn improve

the decision-making process.   Until this is achieved, I would plead
for more understanding and critical interpretation of data obtained
to detect early toxicity.

REFERENCES

1. J. B. Miale, in "Advances in Automated Analysis," Thurman Asso-
    ciates, Miami, 1971, p. 387.

2. M. F. Collen, R. Feldman, A. B. Siegelaub, and D. Crawford, N.
    Engl. J. Med., 283:459 (1970).

3. R. C. Ahlvin, N. Engl. J. Med., 283:1084 (1970).

4. C. E. Boonstra and C. E. Jackson, Ann. Int. Med., 57:963 (1962).

5. D. J. Bryan, J. L. Wearne, A. Viau, A. W. Musser, F. W. Schoon-
    maker, and R. E. Thiers, Clin. Chem., 12:137 (1966).

6. H. E. Paulus, A. Coutts, J. J. Calabro, and J. R. Klinenberg,
    J. Amer. Med. Ass., 211:277 (1970).

Chapter 8

THE USE OF THE EEG
IN INTERPRETING CNS TOXICITY

Simon E. Markovich

University of Miami School of Medicine
and
Mercy Hospital and Variety Children's Hospital
Miami, Florida

In summarizing the role of the clinical researcher, Gibbs has
stated that "The clinical investigator has two responsibilities:
(1) to gain significant information and (2) to convince others of
its significance. Failure to perform the second function reduces
the value of the first (5)."

Basic to the consideration of the electroencephalogram (EEG) as
a useful tool in the evaluation of the effects of drugs in human
beings is the understanding that "normal" EEG is a statistical concept based on the empirical correlation between physiological functions and a structurally normal central nervous system (CNS).

The spontaneous electrical activity of the brain, first described
by Caton in 1875, has become a fascinating objective tool used in
understanding the physiopathology of the CNS. In the past few years
it has helped in studying the pharmacokinetics of many drugs which
have direct or indirect effects on the nervous system. Being a
painless, reproducible test, it has become a fashionable technique
not only in regard to the therapeutic effects of drugs, but in the
relationship between normal and abnormal reactivity of the CNS to
specific medications (4).

It is usually accepted that certain drugs produce CNS depression and/or stimulation. Clinically, depressants are characterized by sedation and sleep, preceded at times by a period of excitement and disinhibition. When given in overdose they may cause coma and death by respiratory failure. Cross-tolerance and cross-dependence has been investigated in most of the drugs of this class, samples of which are the barbiturates, sedatives, and minor tranquilizers.

The second group, the so-called CNS stimulants, are drugs producing excitatory effects characterized by increased wakefulness and alertness and a loss of appetite. In excessive dosage they produce a delirious or psychotic state. The period of excitement or stimulation is usually followed by depression as a rebound phenomenon. Tolerance develops rapidly and is usually accompanied by psychological dependence. This group of drugs includes the amphetamines and cocaine.

Narcotic-analgesic compounds are drugs that relieve pain, induce sedation, and occasionally elevate mood, particularly if it is depressed. A high degree of tolerance and severe psychological dependence usually develop with prolonged or repeated use. Withdrawal symptoms are often uncomfortable. Overdosage causes death by respiratory depression. The most common examples of this variety of drug are opium, morphine, paregoric, codeine, meperidine (Demerol), and methadone (Dolophine). It also includes a variety of so-called analgesic compounds, of which dextropropoxyphene HCl (Darvon) is an example.

The hallucinogens are another important group that has become part of our "new culture," producing toxic effects, delirium, visual illusions and hallucinations accompanied by disturbances in proprioception, paresthesias, and perceptual disorders. Examples of these drugs are LSD (D-lysergic acid diethylamide), mescaline, cannabis (marijuana).

I have listed some of the clinical symptoms to emphasize the overlapping effects of these medications which may confuse the observer, making it difficult to separate them on clinical grounds alone.

It should also be pointed out that the lack of marked individual

differences in the effects of these drugs is equalled by the lack
of sensitive analytical methods to examine them on the basis of conventional laboratory tests. The biological disposition of some of
these drugs cannot be measured on the blood levels. Neither can
their toxic effect on organs, such as the liver, that might have a
profound effect on the metabolism of a given compound (2).

The precise objective measurements of analgesia, for instance,
is very complex. Some subjectivity is always inherent although
double blind procedures can minimize the bias of the patient and/or
the observer. It is sometimes difficult to obtain comparable results even with the same drug, particularly when different groups
of investigators use different evaluative techniques. It is fascinating to recognize, for instance, that pain relief does not correlate with the plasma level of a given drug nor with its excretion
in the urine. It is often difficult to know what the pharmacokinetic mechanism behind the individual differences is and what is
the significance of these differences in terms of drug response (1).

Wikler (6) has proposed a general theory of the relation of EEG
changes to behavioral changes in man. He suggests that "regardless
of the nature of the drug administered, shifts in the patterns of
EEG in the direction of dysyndhronization occur in association with
anxiety, hallucinations, fantasies, illusions or tremors and in the
direction of synchronization in euphoria, relaxation and drowsiness."
This statement stands only in general. In specific cases such as
the paradoxical effects of methylphenidate HCl (Ritalin), in hyper-
kinetic children, or in the group of the so-called non-barbituric
hypnotics (glutethimide (Doriden) and flurazepam HCl (Dalmane)),
it can be easily shown that the clinical effects are different, in
spite of the same typical electrographic patterns.

In conclusion we might say that:

1. EEG is found to be easily recordable and a sensitive and
    quantifiable index of brain functions in studies of human
    pharmacology.

2. The problem of defining and quantifying the EEG is not

difficult if we consider that tests taken at different peaks
in the study of drug effects can be compared to baseline
records.

3. The standard recording in a given individual can be examined
on visual-hand measurements and/or with computerized techniques with electronic frequency analysis when necessary.
In the visual description of the record the state of alertness must be clearly defined to estimate the predominant
rhythms, basic frequencies, symmetry and special types of
waveforms. The record should also include percentage time,
central frequency of various bands, and average voltage (3).

4. In general, drugs that produce the same effect on the EEG
have similar clinical and pharmacological properties.

5. Any studies concerning sleep patterns modified by drugs
should be carefully evaluated, since total understanding of
the physiopathology of sleep is not yet available.

6. Certain drugs introduce important factors like alteration
of the CNS metabolism and cerebral blood flow. Such factors
should be examined carefully in relation to their therapeutic indications and contraindications.

REFERENCES

1. B. Alexanderson and F. Sjoqvist, Ann. N. Y. Acad. Sci., 179:739
   (1971).

2. B. Berkowitz, Ann. N. Y. Acad. Sci., 179:269 (1971).

3. M. Fink, in "EEG and Behavior," ed. Gilbert H. Glaser, Basic
   Books Inc., New York, 1963, p. 177.

4. G. A. Glaser, in "EEG and Behavior," ed. Gilbert H. Glaser,
   Basic Books Inc., New York, 1963.

5. F. A. Gibbs, Electroenceph. Clin. Neurophysiol., 8:149
   (1956).

6. A. Wikler, J. Nerv. Ment. Dis., 120:157 (1954).

7. AMA Drug Evaluations (1971) Library of Congress Catalogue #75-
   147249.

Chapter 9

DETECTION OF OCULAR TOXICITY

Don H. Nicholson

Bascom Palmer Eye Institute
and
Department of Ophthalmology
University of Miami School of Medicine
Miami, Florida

INTRODUCTION

The difficulty of detecting toxic effects of new drugs on the
eye can be appreciated if we first examine the wide range of systemically administered agents which affect the eye and the diversity
of adverse ocular effects which they produce. Table 1 contains an
abbreviated list of the most commonly suspected associations. It
is obvious from this list that we cannot predict which drugs will
affect the eye adversely simply on the basis of systemic pharmacologic effect. Virtually any new drug, or any new dosage regimen of
an old drug, may be associated with adverse ocular effects. Moreover, almost every ocular structure or function may be liable to
toxic effect. A comprehensive monitoring of all possible areas of
toxicity would have to include lid pigmentation; appearance of con-
junctiva; slit-lamp appearance of the cornea and lens; refractive
error and accommodative power; visual acuity and central visual
fields; ophthaloscopic appearance of the optic nerve, vessels and
retina; intraocular pressure; color vision; and ocular motility.

TABLE 1

Adverse Ocular Effects of
Systemically Administered Drugs

Drugs	Adverse Effects
Anticholinergics	Elevated intraocular pressure
Arsenicals	Keratopathy Optic neuropathy
Chloramphenicol	Optic neuropathy
Chloroquine	Retinopathy Accommodative weakness Keratopathy
Chlorpropamide	Optic neuropathy
Corticosteroids	Cataract Pseudotumor cerebri Elevated intraocular pressure
Digitalis	Dyschromatopsia
2, 4-Dinitrophenol	Cataract
Diphenylhydantoin	Conjunctivitis Ophthalmoplegia
Disulfram	Optic neuropathy
Ethambutol	Optic neuropathy
Gold	Blepharoconjunctivitis Keratopathy
Indomethacin	Keratopathy Retinopathy
Isoniazid	Optic neuropathy
Penicillamine	Optic neuropathy
Phenothiazines	Lid pigmentation Keratopathy Cataract Retinopathy Oculogyric crisis
Quinine	Retinopathy Optic neuropathy
Silver	Keratopathy
Sulfonamides	Stevens-Johnson syndrome Acute myopia Optic neuropathy

TABLE 1 (Continued)

Adverse Ocular Effects of
Systemically Administered Drugs

Drugs	Adverse Effects
Triparanol	Cataract
	Blepharitis
Vincristine	Ophthalmoplegia
Vitamin A	Pseudotumor cerebri
Vitamin D	Band keratopathy

SPECIFIC EXAMPLES

In order to illustrate our capabilities and limitations in specific areas of ocular toxicity, I have selected for more detailed
examination three drugs which have been intensively studied in this
respect. These examples permit us to judge how effectively we can
predict or prevent ocular toxicity under optimal circumstances,
that is, once we have identified both the drug and the site of its
adverse ocular effect.

Triparanol (MER-29) Cataracts

Although triparanol is probably the best example we shall ever
have of an unquestionably cataractogenic drug being given to thou-
sands of human beings, we were able to salvage from the triparanol
mass disaster remarkably little scientific knowledge. No attempts
were made to study the epidemiology of drug-induced cataract in
man, and only Kirby (1) collected and published enough retrospective
data to give us a general idea of the clinical features of triparanol cataracts. His data are derived from nine patients whom he
examined at the Mayo Clinic. Only six other similar patients are
described in the literature, so that we are forced to construct our
clinical picture on the basis of fifteen affected patients, when in

fact the total number of patients developing triparanol cataracts
may have been as high as 1500! (2).

The chronologic development of triparanol cataract and the associated dermatologic and ocular findings in Kirby's nine patients
are summarized in Table 2. The duration of therapy preceding the
onset of visual loss, as well as the total daily drug dosage, varied
widely. All patients developing triparanol cataracts in this series
had first experienced the ectodermal side effects (loss and graying
of hair, ichthyosis) which first brought triparanol damage to medical attention. An important feature of triparanol-induced cataracts
which is shared by other cataractogenic agents is the latent interval between drug therapy and the appearance of lens opacities. All
of the adult patients in Kirby's series had a latent interval between cessation of triparanol and appearance of lens opacity which
ranged from a few months to a year or more. The only patient who
did not exhibit this latent interval was a child. Once the lens
opacity appeared, triparanol cataracts characteristically progressed
rapidly and required surgery within several months.

Are there specific morphologic features which enable the ophthalmologist to state whether a given cataract is triparanol-induced?
Careful morphologic descriptions of triparanol cataracts at various

TABLE 2*

Triparanol (MER-29) Cataract

Duration of therapy	1 to 13 months
Daily dosage	125 to 1500 mg
Ectodermal side effects	Present in all patients
Other ocular side effects	5 out of 9 patients
Latent interval	0 to 12 months
Progression period	3 to 9 months

*From Reference 1

stages in their development are too few to answer this question
with certainty, but the morphologic features noted by Kirby are
summarized in Table 3. The crystalline lens is a simple structure
with very limited responses to the insults of drugs, radiation, or
age, and the changes in Table 3 are unlikely to be specific for triparanol cataracts. More importantly for our purpose, the features
noted by Kirby require a much more critical slit-lamp examination
of the lens than ophthalmologists routinely perform. For example,
ophthalmologists frequently perform slit-lamp examination of the
anterior segment of the eye prior to instillation of dilating drops.
If during ophthalmoscopy no lens opacities are noted which interfere
with the red reflex, the slip lamp is not again used to examine the
lens. Many congenital or acquired lens opacities do not interfere
with ophthalmoscopic examination or visual acuity, and many are not
visible when the slit-lamp beam is directed through the undilated
pupil.

In summary, the little we know about triparanol cataracts does
teach some important practical difficulties encountered in the clinical study of potentially cataractogenic drugs (Table 4). First,
there will probably be no unique morphologic features which will

TABLE 3*

Triparanol Cataract: Morphologic Features

Posterior Subcapsular Opacity

    Color gray to yellowish
    Margin irregular, density greatest centrally
    Vacuoles at periphery of main opacity
    Anterior surface irregular with swirled effect
    Rapid increase in density of main opacity

Anterior Subcapsular Opacity

    Fine dusting along suture lines
    Irregularly placed anterior subcapsular vacuoles

---

*From Reference 1

TABLE 4

Difficulties in
Establishing Diagnosis of Drug-Induced Cataract

Pretreatment status unknown

Congenital or developmental opacities
Early senile cataract

Alternative explanations for cataract formation

Underlying disease state
Exposure to other cataractogenic stimuli

Time course of drug-induced cataracts

---

label the opacity as unequivocally drug-induced. Second, in many
cases no pretreatment description of the lens is available. Congenital lens opacities or early senile nuclear sclerosis may be present
in a patient whose visual acuity can be corrected to 20/20, so that
a statement of 20/20 visual acuity prior to institution of drug therapy does not guarantee that lens changes were not present. Third,
the age of the patient, his underlying disease or nutritional status, and exposure to other drugs or irradiation may be an equally
valid explanation for the development of cataracts in a patient
given a new drug. Finally, the latent period between drug therapy
and cataract formation suggests that careful observation should be
continued for at least a year after cessation of the possible cataractogenic agent.

Chloramphenicol Optic Neuropathy

Chloramphenicol is an example of a drug used for many years
without producing ocular side effects. However, when a change in
the dosage and duration of therapy occurred, ocular toxicity was
noted. Thus, even the most exhaustive ophthalmic investigations
during Phase 1 studies or during the first years of its unlimited
clinical use would not have permitted prediction of the effect which
became apparent only after it was given to patients with cystic

fibrosis at therapeutic dose levels for long periods of time.

The clinical picture of chloramphenicol optic neuropathy which emerged after this change in pattern of administration has been delineated by Harley and his associates in a longitudinal study of 98 cystic fibrosis patients receiving long-term chloramphenicol therapy (3). Typically, the affected patients developed an acute loss of visual acuity simultaneously in both eyes after an interval of chloramphenicol therapy ranging from several months to several years. Ocular examination generally disclosed bilateral central scotomas and some optic-disc edema. If chloramphenicol was discontinued, visual acuity returned to normal in the majority of patients, although severe permanent visual loss was noted in approximately 20%. The incidence of chloramphenicol optic neuropathy among the patients observed by Harley et al. (3) did seem related both to daily dosage and duration of therapy (Tables 5 and 6). A second course of chloramphenicol in some instances was associated with a second attack of optic neuropathy which resolved after the drug was discontinued. In other cases, however, a second course of therapy was associated with no recurrence of visual symptoms.

Chloroquine Retinopathy

Chloroquine is another drug which was used initially for many years without any adverse ocular effects, but which, with an

TABLE 5[*]

Chloramphenicol Optic Neuropathy: Relation to Daily Dosage

Daily Dose (mg/kg)	Total No. Pts.	Optic Neuropathy Pts.	Percent
10–25	19	1	5
25–50	71	9	13
Over 50	8	3	38

[*]From Reference 3.

TABLE 6[*]

Chloramphenicol Optic Neuropathy:
Relation to Duration of Therapy

Duration (Months)	Total No. Pts.	Optic Neuropathy Pts.	Percent
Less than 3	11	0	0
3-6	26	3	12
6-12	24	4	16
Over 12	37	6	16

[*]From Reference 3

alteration of dosage schedules, duration of therapy, and nature of patient population, has become our most frequently encountered and intensively studied retinotoxic drug. Serial examinations of large numbers of patients receiving high-dose, long-term chloroquine therapy have provided some general statistics indicating the relationship of total chloroquine dosage and duration of therapy to incidence of retinopathy (Tables 7, 8). In the context of our present discussion, the most instructive investigations of chloroquine retinopathy have been those addressed to its basic definition and early detection. The onset of symptoms is, unlike that in chloramphenicol optic neuropathy, subtle and insidiously progressive. Although the site of ocular toxicity is in the retina, ophthalmoscopic observation has proved a relatively crude means of detection. Early ophthalmoscopic changes are a loss of the foveal reflex and an increased granularity of the retinal pigment epithelium, both of which occur as normal consequences of ageing. Eventually the macular pigment changes progress to form the familiar bull's-eye pattern of normal pigment epithelium in the central macula surrounded by a ring of depigmentation. By the time these extensive pigment changes are noted, visual loss generally cannot be reversed by discontinuing chloroquine. In fact, if the drug is not discontinued before this stage, both visual loss and pigment

TABLE 7[*]

Chloroquine Retinopathy: Relation to Total Dose

Total Dose (grams)	Total No. Pts.	No. Retinopathy Pts.	Percent
Less than 100	46	2	4
100-200	71	9	13
200-300	67	2	3
300-400	74	15	20
400-500	63	9	14
500-600	42	11	26
600-700	12	4	33
700-800	4	2	--
800-900	6	1	--
Over 900	12	7	--
Total	397	62	16

[*]From Reference 4.

epithelial alterations may progress for a variable period after cessation of therapy, with improvement in visual function unlikely.

Clearly the ophthalmoscope is not an adequately sensitive instrument for detecting chloroquine retinal toxicity at a potentially reversible stage. In spite of the intensive application of every known
clinical test of retinal function to patients receiving long-term
chloroquine therapy, no single test has been confirmed as a reliable
detector of impending irreversible retinal toxicity. To be sure, an
altered dark-adaption threshold for red stimuli (5) and a prolonged
recovery time after photostress testing (6) are sensitive enough to
demonstrate the fact that chloroquine does exert a toxic effect on
the retina in virtually <u>all</u> patients who have received a certain minimum total drug dose. However, these tests do not discriminate the
group of patients who will develop clinically significant retinal

TABLE 8[*]

Chloroquine Retinopathy:
Relation to Duration of Therapy

Duration (years)	Total No. Pts.	No. Retinopathy Pts.	Percent
Less than 1	34	1	3
1-2	60	6	10
2-3	73	8	11
3-4	68	11	16
4-5	55	12	22
5-6	61	13	21
6-7	28	7	25
7-9	10	1	30
Over 9	8	1	13
Total	397	62	16

[*]From Reference 4.

damage. The electroretinogram (ERG), electrooculogram (EOG), conventional dark-adaptation thresholds for white light, Amsler grid
testing, color-vision testing, and fluorescein fundus angiography
are other studies which have been applied and, in spite of promising
reports from one or two centers, have been found to be unreliable
early detectors of chloroquine retinopathy at a clinically significant but potentially reversible stage. If other centers confirm
the findings of Percival and Meanock, tangent-screen field testing
with large red rest objects may be the most promising single test
of the many tried. In clinical practice at present, however, we
must combine a statistical generalization concerning safe drug dosage and duration of therapy with periodic eye examination and application of all of the retinal-function tests available at each particular institution, hoping that the statistical guidelines or

abnormalities in one of the function tests will enable us to steer
the difficult course of maintaining drug therapy for as long a period as possible for systemic benefit without ocular jeopardy.

CONCLUSION

The foregoing examples illustrate some of the difficulties encountered in defining ocular toxicities which occur relatively frequently. If adverse ocular effects occur in a much smaller fraction
of patients receiving a drug; if the adverse effects occur only in
patients with a specific preexisting ocular condition; if the time
course of the adverse effect is prolonged, or if a long latent interval between therapy and adverse effect is present, then the probability of recognizing an ocular change as an adverse drug effect
is reduced even further (8).

From a practical standpoint, how can we best screen large numbers of patients for all signs of ocular toxicity? Is it possible
to devise a practical protocol which will permit surveillance not
only for ocular toxicity during preliminary clinical testing of a
new drug, but also for late effects occurring only after treatment
is discontinued or a new regimen of drug administration is introduced?

One approach to early detection of ocular toxicity is to select
a limited number of patients for periodic comprehensive basic ocular
examinations (Table 9). As indicated in the discussion of triparanol
cataract and chloroquine retinopathy, unless very sensitized slit-
lamp and fundus examinations are performed, subtle changes in the
lens or macula may easily be overlooked in this "comprehensive"
screening examination. Its main disadvantage, however, is that the
availability of consultant ophthalmologists and the cost of the
examination make it impractical for all patients given a new drug
to be followed indefinitely by this method. To reduce the cost of
examination and increase the number of ophthalmologists who can contribute, some protocols employ serial examinations by ophthalmology

residents. The obvious disadvantage of this compromise is that the
benefit of observer continuity is lost. Lens changes regarded by
one observer as tiny congenital opacities which do not merit special
mention in the chart may be described by his successor in sufficient
detail that a reviewer might think the opacities had developed during
the interval between the two examinations.

To offset these limitations, ancillary tests of retinal or optic-
nerve function may be included in the protocol (Table 9). These
tests dó provide more detailed information about various visual functions in a given patient, but their limitations in predicting early
toxicity are clearly demonstrated in the instance of chloroquine
retinopathy. One item on the list of ancillary diagnostic tests does
merit special consideration. Serial fundus photographs provide an
objective, permanent record of the appearance of the optic nerve,
vessels, and macula. The quality of the photographs depends upon
the clarity of the cornea, lens, and vitreous, so that a review of
fundus photographs also provides direct evidence about the optical
clarity of these media. The difficulties encountered when several
ophthalmologists examine a patient over the course of time are elim-
inated, since the fundus photographs can be compared by a single
observer who is able to pay particular attention to a specific subtle structural change (e.g., loss of foveal reflex) which might be
omitted from written examination records. In summary, "comprehensive" ophthalmologic evaluation of relatively small numbers of patients enrolled in clinical drug trials is a poor way to screen for
ocular toxicity.

A more effective detection scheme would screen all patients
before and during treatment with a new drug or a new dosage regimen
of a previously approved drug through all phases of drug investigation and for an arbitrary period after the drug is discontinued.
In order to accomplish this objective, provision must be made for
(1) a screening examination protocol to accumulate data on large
patient populations, (2) more comprehensive investigation of patients
in whom abnormalities are detected during the screening examination,

TABLE 9

Detection of Ocular Toxicity: Shotgun Approach

Basic Ocular Examination

    Visual acuity, distance and near
    Refraction
    External appearance
    Pupillary reaction
    Motility
    Confrontation fields
    Intraocular pressure
    Slit lamp examination with dilated pupil
    Fundus examination with dilated pupil

Ancillary Tests for Optic Nerve or Retinal Toxicity

    Visual field testing
        Peripheral fields
        Central fields
        Amsler grid
    Color vision
    Photostress test
    Electroretinography (ERG)
    Electrooculography (EOG)
    Fundus photography
    Fluorescein fundus angiography

---

and (3) a system for review of data collected by screening and comprehensive examinations.

The screening examination protocol is the critical item which determines both the practicality and potential for success of the detection scheme. To assure its applicability to the tremendous number
of patients involved, the screening examination must (1) include only
observations which have the highest probability of detecting ocular
toxicity, (2) minimize cost per patient, (3) generate data which are
amenable to objective recording and review, and (4) completely eliminate physicians (ophthalmologists or otherwise) as screening examin-
ers. One example of such a screening examination would consist of
two basic parts:

1. Visual acuity and ocular history recording. These could be
    done before drug therapy and at 6 to 12 month intervals, most
    easily at the primary physician's office, by placing a Snel-
    len acuity chart in the hall and training the office nurse to
    record visual acuity and ocular history just as she has been
    trained to record the patient's weight and vital signs. Pa-
    tients with less than 20/25 or 20/30 corrected acuity before
    drug treatment and those whose acuity decreased by one Snel-
    len line during the course of follow-up would be sent to a
    consultant ophthalmologist for evaluation. The abbreviated
    history should be structured to detect ocular abnormalities
    which cannot be ascertained from the screening examination
    tests. For example, the patient should be specifically asked
    about symptoms of night blindness, whereas questions about
    central acuity in standard illumination are superfluous, since
    this is determined objectively by acuity recording.

2. Fundus and red reflex photographs, the former preferably
    stereoscopic, should be obtained and incorporated into the
    patient's permanent record prior to institution of drug treat-
    ment and at intervals of 6 to 12 months. These can be ob-
    tained at any university eye clinic at a fraction of the cost
    of a routine eye examination (at our institute, for example,
    the cost of a set of stereoscopic fundus photographs is
    $10.00, whereas the basic private office visit is $35.00
    without pictures). These photographs would provide a per-
    manent record of fundus appearance and alterations in the
    cornea or lens which are prominent enough to interfere with
    the red reflex.

The more comprehensive ocular examination should be performed
by a consultant ophthalmologist only on patients referred from the
screening examination level for evaluation of subnormal visual acuity or from the review level for evaluation of fundus abnormalities
or opacities in the ocular media.

These relatively simple examinations, applied to large numbers
of patients, should provide a more useful data base for tracking down
suspected ocular toxicities than do current protocols for ocular examination during clinical investigation of new drugs. The final part
of the detection program should provide for periodic review of acuity
data and photographs by a consultant ophthalmologist.

Unless a system for recording and reviewing ocular findings in
large study populations is implemented, assumption and anecdote will
continue to exert disproportionate influence on our conclusions concerning postulated relationships between drug administration and
ocular disorders.

REFERENCES

1. T. J. Kirby, Trans. Amer. Ophthalmol. Soc., 65:493 (1967).

2. P. D. Rheingold, Calif. Law Rev., 56:116 (1968).

3. R. D. Harley, N. H. Huang, C. H. Macri, and W. R. Green., Trans.
    Amer. Acad. Ophthalmol. Otolaryngol., 74:1011 (1970).

4. U. Nylander, Acta Ophthalmol. Suppl., 92:1 (1967).

5. R. E. Carr, P. Gouras, and R. D. Gunkel, Arch. Ophthalmol., 75:
    171 (1966).

6. R. E. Carr, P. Henkind, N. Rothfield, and I. M. Siegel, Amer. J.
    Ophthalmol. 66:738 (1968).

7. S. P. B. Percival and I. Meanock, Brit. Med. J., 3:579 (1968).

8. D. H. Nicholson and F. B. Walsh, J. Reprod. Med., 3:37 (1969).

Chapter 10

PHOSPHATIDYLINOSITOL AND THE CARDIAC β-ADRENERGIC RECEPTOR

Gerald S. Levey*

Department of Medicine
University of Miami School of Medicine
Miami, Florida

INTRODUCTION

The actions of many hormones appear to be related to their capacity to increase the activity of the membrane-bound enzyme, adenylate cyclase, which catalyzes the conversion of ATP to adenosine 3',5'-cyclic monophosphate (cyclic AMP). The hormone receptor site in the external surface of the cell is critical in this scheme of hormone action. Current evidence suggests that hormone receptors consist of proteins and phospholipids (1,2). In this regard, we have reported the preparation of a solubilized myocardial adenylate cyclase utilizing a nonionic detergent, Lubrol-PX (3,4). The solubilized myocardial adenylate cyclase in the presence or absence of detergent is unresponsive to the hormones which activate the particulate enzyme, including the catecholamines, isoproterenol, epinephrine and norepinephrine (3). We have studied the role of phosphatidylinositol, as it relates to the catecholamine responsiveness of solubilized myocardial adenylate cyclase, using a preparation freed of detergent by DEAE-cellulose chromatography. The data we have obtained demonstrate

*Investigator, Howard Hughes Medical Institute

that phosphatidylinositol restores the norepinephrine activation
of solubilized myocardial adenylate cyclase.

METHODS

Preparation of Detergent-Free, Solubilized Adenylate Cyclase

Normal cats were anesthetized with pentobarbital, 25 to 35
mg/kg intraperitoneally, and the heart was quickly excised. The
left ventricle was dissected free of endocardium and epicardium
and about 300 mg of muscle was homogenized in 4.5 ml of a cold
solution containing, in final-concentration: sucrose, 0.25 M; Tris
HCl, 10 mM, pH 7.7; Lubrol-PX, 20 mM; and EDTA-magnesium chloride,
1 mM. The homogenate was centrifuged at 12,000 x g for 10 minutes
at 4°C. Approximately 1.3 ml of the 12,000 x g supernatant containing the solubilized myocardial adenylate cyclase and having a
protein concentration of 4 mg/ml was applied to a 1.0 x 12.0 cm
DEAE-cellulose column equilibrated at 4°C in Tris HCl, 10 mM,
pH 7.7. The flow rate was approximately 0.20 ml/min. The column
containing the enzyme was washed with 15 to 20 volumes of Tris HCl,
10 mM, pH 7.7. Adenylate cyclase was eluted with Tris HCl, 1 M,
pH 7.7. The fraction containing adenylate cyclase activity has
been shown to be totally free of detergent using Lubrol-PX labeled
with ^{14}C in the ethylene-oxide moiety (4).

Adenylate Cyclase Assay

Adenylate cyclase was assayed by the method of Krishna, Weiss,
and Brodie (5). The fractions for assay containing 0.025 to
0.05 mg protein in a total volume of 0.06 ml were incubated at
37°C for 5 minutes with ATP, 1.6 mM α-^{32}P-ATP, 2.5 to 3.5 x 10^6
cpm; theophylline 8 mM; Mg Cl_2, 2 mM; Tris HCl, 21 mM, pH 7.7; and
human serum albumin, 0.8 mg/ml. Phosphatidylinositol dispersed in
Tris HCl, 10 mM, pH 7.7, and norepinephrine were added to the
enzyme at 1°C, and to the other components which were at 23°C.

After 5 minutes the incubations were stopped and the ^{32}P-cyclic 3',5'-AMP accumulated was determined as previously described (6).

Preparation of Phospholipids

Phosphatidylinositol (10 mg/ml) were obtained as solutions in $CHCl_3$. The required amount was placed in a 10 x 75 mm glass test tube and the $CHCl_3$ was removed by evaporation with a stream of nitrogen. One ml of Tris-HCl, 10 mM, pH 7.7, was added to the residue and the lipid was dispersed by sonication with a Sonifier Cell Disrupter, Model W185, Branson Sonic Power Company, until there was no apparent change in clarity of the solution, generally one-half to one minute. The phospholipid yielded one spot with thin-layer chromatography in either of two separate solvent systems; either $CHCl_3:CH_3OH:CH_3COOH:H_2O$ (100:60:16:8), or $CHCl_3:CH_3OH:H_2O$ (65:25:4).

MATERIALS

Chromatographically pure monophosphatidylinositol was prepared from bovine brain by Dr. S. Ramachandran, Applied Science Laboratories, State College, Pennsylvania. L-norepinephrine bitartrate was from Sigma Chemical Co., St. Louis, Missouri. D,L-propranolol was from Ayerst Laboratories, New York. Lubrol-PX was a gift from ICI America, Inc., Stamford, Connecticut. Alpha-labeled ^{32}P-ATP was from International Chemical and Nuclear Corp., Irvine, California.

RESULTS

We have previously demonstrated that phosphatidylserine re-stored the responsiveness of the solubilized myocardial adenylate cyclase to histamine and glucagon (7,8). However, phosphatidyl-serine did not restore responsiveness to the catecholamines. Another acidic phospholipid, phosphatidylinositol, restored

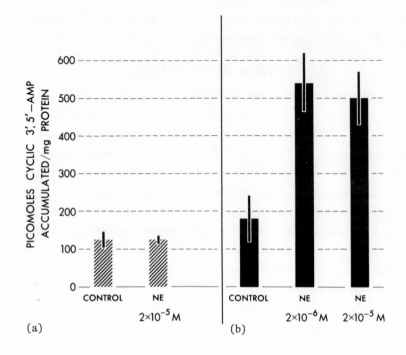

FIG. 1. Effect of phosphatidylinositol on hormone responsiveness of solubilized myocardial adenylate cyclase. Each value
represents the mean ± S.E. of 10 to 23 samples.

responsiveness to norepinephrine (Fig. 1), but did not restore
responsiveness to glucagon or histamine. Norepinephrine activated
the solubilized adenylate cyclase in the presence of phosphatidylinositol over the concentration range $5 \times 10^{-8}M$ to $1 \times 10^{-5}M$,
half-maximal activation occurring at a concentration of norepinephrine, $8 \times 10^{-8}M$. The sensitivity of adenylate cyclase to
norepinephrine in this system as judged by threshold- and
concentration-producing half-maximal activation was approximately
100 times greater than that observed in particulate preparations
(6) and similar to that observed in physiologic preparations.

TABLE 1

Effect of Propranolol (1×10^{-6}M) on the
Norepinephrine Activation of Solubilized Adenylate Cyclase[a]

	Picomoles cyclic 3',5'-AMP accumulated/5 min/mg protein	
	drug absent	drug present
Control	700 ± 175	825 ± 30
Norepinephrine	2400 ± 200	1050 ± 100

[a]Each value represents the mean ± S.E. of four samples.

Effect of D,L-Propranolol on the Norepinephrine-Mediated Activation of Adenylate Cyclase

In order to determine the receptor specificity of this re-constituted system we examined the effect of the β-adrenergic blocking drug, D,L-propranolol on the catecholamine activation. Table 1 shows that D,L-propranolol, 1×10^{-6}M, abolished the activation of adenylate cyclase produced by 2×10^{-6}M norepinephrine. Similar findings have been reported for the particulate enzyme (9).

Effective Concentrations of Phosphatidylinositol

Phosphatidylinositol, 0.05 μg/incubation (0.8 μg/ml) was half-maximally effective in restoring norepinephrine responsiveness. Concentrations of phosphatidylinositol less than 0.025 μg/incubation (0.4 μg/ml) were ineffective and those greater than 0.25 μg/incubation (4 μg/ml) were maximally effective.

Binding of Norepinephrine to Solubilized Myocardial Adenylate Cyclase

In order to define the site of phospholipid action and to determine whether or not phospholipids are required for binding, we examined the binding of 7-^{3}H-D,L-norepinephrine in this solubilized preparation. Table 2 shows that binding of

TABLE 2

Binding of 7-^{3}H-D,L-Norepinephrine to
Solubilized Myocardial Adenylate Cyclase[a]

7-^{3}H-D,L-norepinephrine (M)	Picomoles 7-^{3}H-D,L-norepinephrine bound/60 min/mg protein
0	--
1×10^{-8}	2
1×10^{-7}	20
1×10^{-6}	150
5×10^{-6}	650
1×10^{-5}	620

[a]Each value represents the mean ± S.E. of 3-6 samples.

norepinephrine occurs in the absence of added phospholipid. This
data is in agreement with the data of Lefkowitz and Levey, which
showed that half-maximal displacement of bound 7-^{3}H-D,L-norepine-
phrine is the same either in the presence or absence of phospholipid (10).

DISCUSSION

A large body of evidence has accumulated which emphasizes the
importance of phospholipids in hormone-sensitive adenylate cyclase
systems. Solubilized preparations of adenylate cyclase from brain,
heart, skeletal muscle, and liver are unresponsive to the hormones
which activate the membrane-bound enzyme (11,12). In addition,
certain phospholipases decrease the effects of hormones on their
target tissues (12-14) and decrease the binding of glucagon to
isolated liver membranes (15). Pohl and coworkers reported that
addition of pure phosphatidylserine partially restored glucagon
responsiveness of adenylate cyclase in phospholipase-A-treated
liver membranes and the binding of glucagon to these membranes
(15).

The data in this report demonstrate that phosphatidylinositol selectively restores responsiveness of the solubilized myocardial adenylate cyclase to the catecholamines. A marked increase in sensitivity was noted for norepinephrine in the presence of phosphatidylinositol as compared to concentration response curves noted with the particulate enzyme and norepinephrine (6). The degree of sensitivity in the reconstituted system approaches that found in intact physiologic preparations (16). The reason for this striking increase in sensitivity is obscure, but suggests that the process of homogenization alone alters the lipid-enzyme relationship, resulting in decreased sensitivity of the enzyme to hormonal stimulation in particulate preparations.

It is of great interest that phosphatidylinositol not only restored catecholamine responsiveness of solubilized adenylate cyclase, but β-adrenergic-receptor specificity was retained as well. This was clearly shown by the results with D,L-propranolol, a specific β-adrenergic blocking agent which abolished the activation of adenylate cyclase by norepinephrine in the presence of phosphatidylinositol. These data concerning receptor specificity would appear to add greater significance to this in vitro system in terms of its usefulness in understanding the molecular components which compose these cardiac β-adrenergic hormone receptors in vivo.

The precise site and mechanism of action of the phospholipid is unclear. These phospholipids may induce a specific conformational change in the enzyme molecule necessary for binding of the hormone and subsequent activation of the enzyme.

According to current concepts of the membrane-bound adenylate cyclase, it is considered to be a three-component system (17). The total unit consists of a regulatory site, a catalytic site and an intermediate coupler. The regulatory site, which faces the external surface of the membrane, discriminates between hormones and serves as the binding site of hormone to target membrane. The catalytic site faces the interior surface of the membrane, has access to ATP and generates the cyclic 3',5'-AMP. An intermediate

unit or coupler serves to transmit a signal from the regulatory
site to the catalytic site. The catalytic site can be directly
activated by sodium fluoride and appears to be independent of
lipid since fluoride activation of the solubilized adenylate
cyclase is unimpaired, whereas hormone activation is absent
(3,11,15). The regulatory site of the cardiac enzyme also is
largely independent of phospholipid, since binding occurs in the
absence or presence of lipid in an equivalent manner. Thus it
would seem that the major site of action of phospholipid is the
coupler site. These data also provide a clear dissociation of the
process of binding of hormone to receptors and the activation of
adenylate cyclase.

SUMMARY

Several investigations have demonstrated that phospholipids
play an important role in hormone-sensitive adenylate-cyclase
systems. Particulate preparations of myocardial adenylate cyclase
are activated by glucagon, histamine, and norepinephrine whereas
solubilized preparations are not. The addition of certain phospholipids restored the hormone responsiveness of solubilized
myocardial adenylate cyclase. Phosphatidylserine restored the
activation produced by glucagon and histamine but not norepinephrine. As shown in this report, phosphatidylinositol restored
responsiveness to norepinephrine but not to glucagon or histamine.
Sensitivity of the solubilized adenylate cyclase to norepinephrine
in the presence of phosphatidylinositol was increased almost
100-fold compared to particulate preparations. The β-adrenergic
blocking agent, D,L-propranolol, abolished the norepinephrine
activation. The site and mechanism of action of these lipids is
unclear, but they probably act on the coupler site between the
receptor and catalytic sites, producing the necessary molecular
configuration of the enzyme for specific hormone activation.

ACKNOWLEDGMENTS

This investigation was supported in part by United States Public Health Service Grant 1 R01 HE13715-03 and the Heart Association of Broward County, a chapter of the Florida Heart Association.

The author is grateful to Mrs. Eva Ruiz and Mrs. Antoinette Schenk for their excellent technical assistance.

REFERENCES

1. D. R. Waud, Pharmacol. Rev., 20: 49 (1968).

2. S. Ehrenpreis, J. H. Fleish, and T. W. Mittag, Pharmacol. Rev., 21: 131 (1969).

3. G. S. Levey, Biochem. Biophys. Res. Commun., 38: 86 (1970).

4. G. S. Levey, Ann. N.Y. Acad. Sci., 185: 449 (1971).

5. G. Krishna, B. Weiss, and B. B. Brodie, J. Pharmacol. Exp. Ther., 163: 379 (1968).

6. G. S. Levey, C. L. Skelton, and S. E. Epstein, J. Clin. Invest., 48: 2244 (1969).

7. G. S. Levey, Biochem. Biophys. Res. Commun., 43: 108 (1971).

8. G. S. Levey and I. Klein, J. Clin. Invest., 51: 1578 (1972).

9. G. S. Levey and S. E. Epstein, Clin. Res., 24: 151 (1969).

10. R. J. Lefkowitz and G. S. Levey, Life Sci., 2: 821 (1972).

11. E. W. Sutherland, T. W. Rall, and T. Menon, J. Biol. Chem., 237: 1220 (1962).

12. L. Birnbaumer, S. L. Pohl, and M. Rodbell, J. Biol. Chem., 246: 1857 (1971)

13. M. Rodbell, H. M. J. Krans, S. L. Pohl, and L. Birnbaumer, J. Biol. Chem., 246: 1861 (1971).

14. V. Macchia and I. Pastan, J. Biol. Chem., 242: 1864 (1967).

15. S. L. Pohl, H. M. J. Krans, V. Kozyreff, L. Birnbaumer, and M. Rodbell, J. Biol. Chem., 246: 4447 (1971).

16. R. A. Buccino, J. F. Spann, Jr., P. E. Pool, E. H. Sonnenblick, and E. Braunwald, J. Clin. Invest., 45: 1669 (1967).

17. M. Rodbell, L. Birnbaumer, and S. L. Pohl, in "The role of
     adenyl cyclase and cyclic 3',5'-AMP in biological systems,"
     eds. T. W. Rall, M. Rodbell, and P. G. Condliffe. Government
     Printing Office, Washington, D.C., 1971, p. 59.

Chapter 11

MODE OF ACTIVATION OF ADENYLYL CYCLASES BY
RECEPTORS AND ITS REGULATION BY NUCLEOTIDES AND NUCLEOSIDES

Lutz Birnbaumer

Department of Cell Biology
Baylor College of Medicine
Houston, Texas 77025

The discriminating (or hormone recognizing) function of a hormone receptor, as well as its function in initiating an effect
(coupling-signal-generating function) can be explored by studying
hormonal stimulation of the adenylyl-cyclase system, making these
functions useful models for the study of the mode of action of hormone receptors in cell-free systems. In addition, the discrimina-
tory function of hormone receptors can be explored more directly
by studying the specific binding of labeled hormone to receptor-
containing materials and correlating this phenomenon with the
effects of receptor occupation seen by determining adenylyl-cyclase
activity. Studies of this sort have in recent years yielded much
new information about the mechanism of action of peptide and protein
hormones and have revealed the existence of regulatory processes,
dependent on phospholipids and on nucleotides, which were previously
unknown.

In the article that follows we shall review some of these
findings. First, we shall analyze the characteristics of hormone
receptors in intact cells and in cell-free systems, and evaluate,
based on the experimental evidence at hand, whether or not isolated

93

membrane systems are adequate for studying the receptor functions.
Second, we shall analyze the utility and restrictions of hormone-
binding studies, and evaluate their meaning, taking into consideration independent information gained from studies with adenylyl-
cyclase systems. Third, we shall discuss what we know about the
so-called coupling process intervening between receptor occupation
and adenylyl-cyclase activation. It will be shown that this process
is under, both positive and negative regulation by nucleotides,
especially GTP and ATP, and that adenylyl-cyclase activation is
therefore not simply a passive, receptor-dependent phenomenon.
Rather, it is under the constant regulatory influence of cell
metabolism, be it normal or modified by other hormones or disease.

CHARACTERISTICS OF ADENYLYL CYCLASE ACTIVATION IN INTACT CELLS

The ultimate test of the physiological significance of properties of cell-free systems is whether these properties are similar
to those observed with intact cells. Accordingly, the hormonal
response of adenylyl cyclases in cell-free systems should exhibit
the same specificity and similar dose-response relationships and
kinetics as seen in intact cells. The characteristics of the
glucagon-stimulated adenylyl-cyclase system in intact liver have
been explored by Miller, Exton and others (1-6), by measuring either
cyclic AMP levels or the cellular effect of cyclic AMP on glyco-
genesis. They have shown that—

1. Among several peptides tested, only glucagon affects the
    system. Secretin, structurally very similar to glucagon
    (7), does not stimulate cyclic-AMP production; and des-1-
    histidine glucagon (DH-glucagon), is inactive in producing
    hyperglycemia in the dog (8,9).

2. The range of concentration over which glucagon acts to in-
    crease intracellular levels of cyclic AMP in the perfused
    liver is 5×10^{-11} to about 10^{-7}M.

3. Allowing for the diffusion of the hormone to the liver cells
    the effects of glucagon on cyclic-AMP production seem to

be established very rapidly with no significant lag before
achieving maximal rates.

4. Administration of glucagon followed by withdrawal results
   in a rapid fall in cyclic-AMP levels in the perfused liver;
   half-maximal levels are observed within 4 minutes of withdrawal (2). The fall in cyclic-AMP levels reflects mainly
   the rate of decay of adenylyl-cyclase activity to its resting state. The rate of cyclic-AMP hydrolysis by phosphodiesterase is not affected by glucagon administration or
   withdrawal. Hence, glucagon-receptor complex formation
   appears to be rapid and reversible.

Thus, in the intact cell, the receptor is specific for a hormone, responds to the hormone over a well-defined concentration
range, and is rapidly and reversibly activated by the hormone.
These properties should persist in cell-free preparations.

CHARACTERISTICS OF ADENYLYL CYCLASE ACTIVATION IN CELL-FREE SYSTEMS

Specificity of Dose-Response Relationships

Addition of glucagon to isolated liver-plasma membranes results
in an 8- to 10-fold stimulation of adenylyl-cyclase activity. This
effect is specific for native glucagon, since secretin, and a great
number of other peptide and protein hormones, including the biologically inactive glucagon derivative, DH-glucagon, were found to be
ineffective stimulators of adenylyl-cyclase activity in isolated
membranes (10,11). In close agreement with liver-perfusion studies,
half-maximal activation of adenylyl cyclase in isolated membranes
is obtained at about 10^{-9}M, varying somewhat with the incubation
conditions. Thus, while Pohl et al. (10) found an apparent activation constant (K_a) for glucagon of 4×10^{-9}M, Lin et al. (12) recently reported an apparent K_a of about 7×10^{-10}M, obtained by
using the synthetic substrate, AMP-PNP, GTP and omitting chelating
agents from the incubation medium—factors shown to modify hormonal
stimulation in isolated adenylyl-cyclase systems. DH-glucagon is
ineffective in stimulating the liver adenylyl-cyclase system;

however, it is a potent <u>inhibitor</u> of glucagon action (11), with an
apparent dissociation constant of about 2 to 4 x 10^{-8}M. DH-glucagon
was found to inhibit glucagon activation of adenylyl cyclase not
only in liver, but also in fat cells and a β-cell tumor of the
Syrian hamster. These results indicate that even though the dis-
criminatory function of the receptor is little affected by the
absence of histidine, initiation of action is absolutely dependent
on its presence; this characteristic being similar in several
tissues (11,13). The dose-response relations for glucagon action
in the intact liver cells and for glucagon action on adenylyl cyclase in isolated liver membranes have therefore been shown to
correlate well. Similarly, epinephrine was found to elevate cyclic-
AMP levels in the rat heart (14) over the same concentration range
that it stimulated adenylyl-cyclase activity in heart homogenates
(15).

    These results illustrate that in some instances hormone-receptor
function is completely preserved upon partial isolation. In other
instances, however, a distinct divergence of the dose-response
curves obtained with intact cells on cyclic-AMP levels and with
isolated membranes on adenylyl-cyclase activity was found. For
example, while ACTH and epinephrine effect cyclic-AMP levels in
isolated rat-fat cells with an apparent K_a of 5 x 10^{-10}M, and
5 x 10^{-8}M respectively (16), in isolated-membrane preparations these
hormones stimulate adenylyl cyclase half-maximally at 3 x 10^{-7}, and
5 x 10^{-6} respectively (17).

    Several possibilities may account for these discrepancies:

1. The membrane system may have been damaged during isolation,
    so that it no longer reflects the physiologic state that
    predominates in the intact cell. Since phospholipids have
    been demonstrated to play a specific role in the coupling
    process, it is likely that such damage might be due to
    alterations (oxidation?) of membrane phospholipids.

2. The intact cell system may have a hormone-concentrating de-
    vice that locally increases hormone concentration and that

has become inoperative in the isolated membrane. Experimentally, this device should consist of hormone-specific
binding sites of high affinity present in large amounts on
the cell surface. The advantage for the cell of having
such a mechanism is that it would aid in assuring that hormones, which circulate at very low levels in blood, "find"
the extremely low number of receptors present on the surface.

3. Non-linear coupling processes may intervene between hormone-
   receptor-complex formation and stimulation of adenylyl
   cyclase.

4. The coupling process may be under the regulatory control of
   soluble metabolites lost or washed out during preparation
   of adenyl-cyclase-containing membranes. This possibility
   is suggested by the recent discovery that purine nucleosides and nucleotides modify hormonal stimulation of
   adenylyl-cyclase systems (18-21).

5. Finally, the shift of the dose-response relationship in
   broken-cell preparations towards higher concentrations may
   be due either to (a) an incubation artifact such as the
   presence of membrane-associated hormone-degrading mechanisms
   whose effect would be noticeable at subsaturating hormone
   concentrations, or (b) to erroneous experimental design,
   such as not allowing enough time for the receptor-binding
   reaction to reach equilibrium before adenylyl-cyclase activity resulting from hormone-receptor interaction is determined. Numerous hormone-binding studies have shown that it
   may take as long as 15 to 20 minutes at 30 to 37° to achieve
   maximal levels of binding (22-27).

Kinetic Aspects of Adenylyl-Cyclase Activation

Looking at data from liver-perfusion experiments, stimulation
of the liver-membrane adenylyl-cyclase system by glucagon is rapid,
as long as saturating concentrations of the hormone are used. The
activation rate at submaximal concentrations, however, depends on

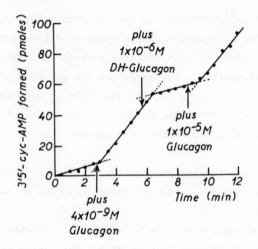

Fig. 1   Time course of cyclic–AMP production by liver-plasma
membranes before and after successive addition of 4 x 10^{-9}M glucagon, 1 x 10^{-6}M des-1-histidine glucagon (DH-glucagon) and 1 x 10^{-5}M
glucagon. Liver membranes were incubated for adenylyl-cyclase
activity in a final volume of 1.3 ml in a 13 x 100 mm test tube at
30°C. Final composition of the incubation medium was: 3.2 mM
$[\alpha-^{32}P]$ATP (approximately 65 cpm/M, 5 mM $MgCl_2$, 1.0 mM cyclic AMP,
1.0 mM EDTA, 20 mM creatine phosphate, 1 mg/ml creatine kinase, and
25 mM Tris HCl, pH 7.5. Test tube and reagents were temperature
equilibrated before initiation of the reaction. Formation of
cyclic AMP was followed by removing 50-µl aliquots and terminating
the reaction by adding them to 100 µl of 40 mM ATP, 12.5 mM $[^3H]$
cyclic AMP (approximately 10,000 cpm) and 1% sodium dodecyl sul-
phate followed by immediate boiling for 3.5 minutes. $[^{32}P]$ cyclic
AMP formed from $[\alpha-^{32}P]$ATP was determined by the method of Krishna
et al. (47). (From Ref. 28.)

the incubation conditions. With high concentrations of ATP, the

presence of EDTA and an ATP-regenerating system, there is no signi-

lag period between hormone addition and attainment of the stimula-

ted state (Fig. 1). However, by modifying the indubation condi-

tions (0.1 mM AMP-PNP, no EDTA, no ATP-regenerating system or GTP)

Lin et al. (12) showed a lag period varying from about 30 seconds

at 10^{-7}M to as much as 4 minutes at 5 x 10^{-10}M. Addition of GTP

significantly reduced this lag time, especially at the low glucagon

concentration, and simultaneously increased the magnitude of acti-

vation.

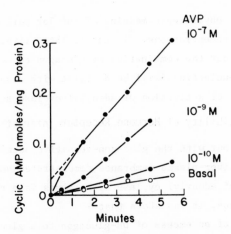

Fig. 2. Time course of cyclic-AMP production by beef renal
medullary membranes and various concentrations of 8-arginine vasopressin (AVP). Beef renal medullary membranes, collected from the
37/41.5% sucrose interface of a discontinuous sucrose-density gradient (from bottom to top: 10 ml 41.5% sucrose, 7.5 ml 37% sucrose,
5 ml 32.5% sucrose and 15 ml of a suspension of 1500 x g particles
prepared from a homogenate of beef renal medulla) after a 2-hour
centrifugation at 27,000 rpm in a Beckman SW 27 rotor, were incubated at 37°C in a final volume of 0.05 ml of medium containing
0.08 mM $[\alpha\text{-}^{32}P]$ATP (2500 cpm/M), 2.0 mM $MgCl_2$, 1.4 mM EDTA, 1.0 mM
cyclic AMP, 20 mM creatine phosphate, 0.2 mg/ml of creatine kinase,
25 mM bis-tris-propane-HCl buffer (Sigma) at pH 8.0, and the indicated concentrations of AVP. Test tubes containing all the ingre-
dients for the assay were "preincubated" for 1 minute at 37°C prior
to the addition of membranes (20-µl aliquots) with which the
reaction was started. At the indicated times the reaction was
stopped by addition of 100 µl of medium containing 40 mM ATP, 10 mM
$[^{3}H]$cyclic AMP (approximately 10,000 cpm) and 1% sodium dodecyl
sulfate followed by boiling for 3.5 minutes. $[^{32}P]$cyclic AMP
formed from $[\alpha\text{-}^{32}]$ATP was determined by the method of Krishna et
al. (47).

This lag period of adenylyl cyclase is not unique to liver

tissue. Bockaert et al. (27) recently reported slow activation of

the adenylyl-cyclase system from pig renal medulla with low con-

centrations of lysinevasopressin (LVP). We have observed a similar

phenomenon working with an arginine-vasopressin(AVP)-sensitive

adenylyl-cyclase system from beef renal medulla when tested at

10^{-10}M and 10^{-9}M AVP (Fig. 2). As yet no definite judgement can be made as to the physiologic meaning of the lag periods observed at low hormonal concentrations. In the isolated liver-plasma membranes it seems that the combination of glucagon concentration and availability of nucleotides will be decisive with respect to the rapidity of onset of activation of adenylyl-cyclase systems.

Reversibility of Hormone Receptor Interaction

Work carried out with the glucagon-sensitive adenylyl-cyclase system from rat-liver-plasma membranes demonstrated unequivocally that activation of adenylyl cyclase by hormones is a reversible process (28). Thus, it was shown that--

1. Addition of an excess of DH-glucagon to a glucagon-stimulated adenylyl-cyclase system proceeding at its half-maximal rate results, within one minute, in the return to basal levels of activity (Fig. 1).

2. Removal of glucagon by washing results in loss of the activated state of the enzyme, provided the concentrations of the peptide hormone to which the membranes were first exposed does not exceed the apparent K_a by more than ten times (23).

3. Dilation of the incubation medium in which glucagon-stimulated adenylyl cyclase is proceeding at a given submaximal rate with glucagon-free incubation medium results in immediate and proportional loss of the stimulated rate of cyclic-AMP production.

4. Submaximally stimulated glucagon activities decay as a function of incubation time, i.e., they are curvilinear, possibly due to significant inactivation of glucagon by a glucagon-specific degrading system present in liver-plasma membranes (22,30).

These studies indicate that adenylyl cyclase is activated reversibly. The proportion of the enzyme in the stimulated state depends on the instantaneous concentration of free hormone in the medium, and by inference, on the proportion of hormone-receptor complex.

With less purified membrane systems (fat-cell ghosts and ACTH, low-speed particles from rat liver and glucagon) higher hormone concentrations resulted in persistent stimulation of adenylyl-cyclase activity which would not be reversed by simple washing procedures (31,32). A similar result was obtained with purified liver-plasma membranes when high concentrations of glucagon (approximately 500 times apparent K_a) were used (29). It is likely that the observed persistent effects are due to binding of the respective hormones to nonspecific sites on the membrane preparations, which upon subsequent incubation, release saturating amounts of the hormone.

The following may therefore be concluded about cell-free studies:

1. The characteristics of adenylyl-cyclase systems in the isolated state may, in some instances, be very close if not identical to the characteristics of these systems in the intact cell.

2. The isolated systems may contain functional receptors with respect to affinity and specificity and to initiation of hormone action.

3. Studies on the mode of action of receptors in the isolated system will lead us to an understanding of the primary events in hormone action, provided the particular system under study has been validated with respect to hormone specificity, dose-response relation, and kinetics.

Hormone Binding; Relation to Adenylyl Cyclase Activation

Rodbell and collaborators (10,11,22,28,30,33,34) carried out an extensive study of the properties of binding of glucagon to specific binding sites in rat-liver-plasma membranes and correlated their results with the characteristics of the receptor-dependent stimulation of adenylyl-cyclase activity.

Binding of biologically active iodinated glucagon to liver-plasma membranes has two main characteristics: (1) it is specific

for glucagon or DH-glucagon; no other peptide or protein hormone
tested interferes with glucagon, and (2) binding occurs in the same
concentration range over which glucagon activates the adenylyl-
cyclase system.

With respect to rapidity and reversibility, however, the binding appears to be complex, and its relation to adenylyl-cyclase
activation is not clear. First, binding is slow, taking about ten
to fifteen seconds to reach constant values at 4×10^{-9}M glucagon.
Second, as the binding reaction proceeds it is associated with a
progressive loss of reversibility. Addition of chase quantities
of unlabeled glucagon 1 minute after initiation of the binding
reaction resulted in the total release (dissociation) of labeled
glucagon from the membranes in one or two minutes. But, a glucagon
chase at 5 and 15 minutes results in rapid release of only about
30% and 10% of the label respectively, the rest being bound almost
irreversibly. This time-dependent loss of reversibility of binding
is overcome by the addition of micromolar concentrations of GTP and
GDP or of millimolar concentrations of ATP. Thus, in the presence
of 10^{-6}M GTP, addition of a glucagon chase after 15 minutes leads
to total dissociation of the label within a few minutes. Finally,
even in the presence of GTP or ATP to assure reversible binding,
the binding reaction does not seem to proceed fast enough to account
for the rapid activation of the receptor-coupled adenylyl-cyclase
system. For example, it was found that in the presence of 1 mM
EDTA, 3.2 mM ATP, and ATP-regenerating system, stimulation of the
adenylyl cyclase by 4×10^{-9}M glucagon is achieved within 10 to 20
seconds, but occupation of the glucagon-specific binding sites is
only 10 to 20% of that achieved with prolonged incubation. In
addition, DH-glucagon, added 5 minutes after glucagon, completely
inhibited hormonal stimulation within one minute, while displacing
only 10 to 20% of the glucagon from its binding sites. This cannot
be reconciled with the receptor-occupation theory of hormone action,
according to which adenylyl-cyclase activation should be proportional to hormone-occupied binding sites.

Such results seem to indicate that a large proportion of the glucagon-specific sites (at least 80 to 90%) do not participate in the activation of the adenylyl-cyclase system and might therefore be related to degrading or concentrating functions. Specific inactivation of glucagon, unrelated to the mechanism of adenylyl-cyclase activation, has been described in liver membranes. Correlative phenomena will have to be carefully considered before non-activating hormone building can be interpreted. For example, there are indications of interaction (cooperativity) between glucagon-specific binding sites, suggested by the finding that more labeled glucagon dissociates in the presence of a glucagon chase than in the presence of a saturating DH-glucagon chase (29,35). Furthermore, results obtained in hormone-sensitive adenylyl-cyclase systems from several tissues (e.g., rat liver, beef renal medulla and cat heart) indicate that translation of the coupling signal, generated by hormone-receptor interaction, into enzyme activation may have several slow components.

Examples of slow reactions were found both in rat liver and beef renal adenylyl cyclase. Thus, in the liver-membrane system with low glucagon concentrations, a considerable lag between initiation of binding and adenylyl-cyclase activation exists if the system is tested under nucleotide-limiting conditions without chelating agents (12). Stimulation of the beef renal medullary membrane adenylyl cyclase by $10^{-7}M$ AVP is superimposed on a "burst" phase (initial velocity greater than steady-state velocity), indicating an initial transient state of activity that is more active than the final steady state of activity (Fig. 2). Such burst phases, although not specifically commented on, have been reported in the data for fluoride-stimulated activity in rat testicular adenylyl-cyclase preparations by Murad et al. (36), for basal adenylyl-cyclase activity in membranes of a β-cell tumor by Goldfine et al. (13) and for both basal and ACTH-stimulated activities in first-cell membranes by Harwood et al. (37). This transient state of activity may be a general phenomenon which has not

yet received enough attention. The existence of lag and burst
phases clearly preclude any simple correlations between the time-
course of hormone binding and the time-course of hormone-dependent
enzyme activation. Activation must be the resultant of a slow (lag
generating), hormone-binding function and a complex, unexplained
burst-generating function, possibly depending on isomerization
processes of the catalytic units of these systems (38,39). It is
conceivable that at a given hormone concentration and in the presence of substances such as nucleotides and/or chelating agents,
these two phenomena "cancel" themselves, yielding "linear" time
curves.

In conclusion, hormone-binding studies are just beginning and
not always comprehensible. In the one study (35) that compared
binding to function, specificity and apparent affinity parameters
correlated well with that required for receptor activity. However,
it appears that a large proportion of specific binding, perhaps as
much as 80 to 90%, is not related to adenylyl-cyclase activation.

The significance of hormone binding which is apparently not
coupled to adenylyl-cyclase activation has yet to be explained.

FACTORS AFFECTING THE COUPLING OF HORMONE-RECEPTOR INTERACTION TO ADENYLYL CYCLASE ACTIVATION

Role of Phospholipids in Coupling

Hormone-sensitive adenylyl-cyclase systems are firmly bound to
plasma membranes and to cells. Many of the properties of these complex multimolecular systems are, therefore, conditioned by the
environment in which they are located. Rodbell, et al., found that
treatment of fat-cell ghosts with phospholipase A resulted in total
loss of enzymatic activity. However, treatment with lower concentrations of phospholipase A resulted in a selective loss of the
responsiveness of the liver system to glucagon, with either unimpaired or stimulated fluoride-sensitive activity. Selective loss
of hormonal stimulation also resulted when liver membranes were
treated with digitonin (40,34). Glucagon stimulation could be

partially restored by the addition of membrane phospolipids or pure

phosphatidyl choline, phosphatidyl ethanolamine, or phosphatidyl

serine (the most effective) (34). These results suggested that

adenylyl cyclases, in addition to being dependent on membrane in-

tegrity, are dependent on phospholipids. This was the first indi-

rect evidence of a selective role of phospholipids in hormonal

stimulation of adenylyl-cyclase systems.

Levey, working with cat-heart adenylyl-cyclase systems provided

further evidence for a specific role of phospholipids in hormonal

response. In a series of elegant experiments (41-43), he demon-

strated that treatment of heart adenylyl cyclase with the non-ionic

degergent, Lubrol-PX, results in loss of the enzyme's response to

norepinephrine and glucagon, and that specific phospholipids re-

store response to either one or the other hormone. Thus, addition

of phosphatidyl inositol selectively restored the response to the

catecholamine and addition of phosphatidyl serine restored response

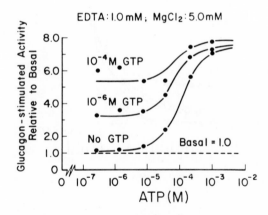

Fig. 3.   Effect of ATP and GTP on stimulation of liver-plasma
membrane adenylyl-cyclase activity by 5 μm glucagon. Activities
in the presence of glucagon were determined in the absence and the
presence of 10^{-6}M and 10^{-4}M GTP. Activities relative to basal were
calculated by dividing the activity obtained in the presence of
glucagon at each ATP concentration by the respective activity
obtained in the absence of glucagon. Incubations were for 2 minutes at 30°C. Other incubation conditions were same as those for
Figure 1.

to glucagon.   (For further details see Levey's article in this
book.)

The Role of Nucleotides and Nucleosides in the Coupling Process

Studies on glucagon binding led Rodbell and collaborators to
study the glucagon-stimulated adenylyl cyclase using the synthetic
substrate, AMP-PNP (19,44), or very low concentrations of ATP (28)
that do not affect the reversibility of binding.   It was found that
under either one of these conditions glucagon-stimulated adenylyl-
cyclase activity is strongly dependent on the addition of low concentrations (10^{-8} to 10^{-6}M) of GTP or relatively high concentrations

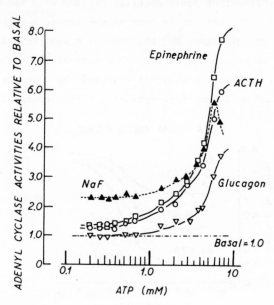

Fig. 4.   Effect of ATP on stimulation of fat-cell "ghost"
adenylyl-cyclase activity by ACTH, glucagon, epinephrine and NaF.
Fat-cell ghosts (for details of preparation see Reference 58) were
incubated in final volume of 0.05 ml for 10 minutes at 30°C with
the indicated concentrations of ATP in the absence (basal) and the
presence of 10 µg/ml ACTH, 10 µg/ml glucagon, 10 µg/ml epinephrine
and 10 mM NaF.   Remaining incubation conditions were: 5 mM $MgCl_2$,
10 mM theophyllin, 0.05% albumin, 10 mM creatine phosphate, 0.2
mg/ml creatine kinase, and 25 mM Tris HCl (pH 7.5).   At each ATP
concentration the stimulation of cyclic-AMP production was expressed relative to that obtained under basal conditions.

(10^{-5} to 10^{-3}M) of ATP (Fig. 3). The concentration range over
which these two nucleotides promote glucagon stimulation is the
same as that over which they promote reversibility of binding. The
extremely low concentration of GTP that affected this system suggested that the guanyl nucleotide and not the adenylyl nucleotide
is the natural effector. GMP-PCP, a nonphosphorylating analogue
of GTP, was also effective in enhancing glucagon stimulation (18).
It seems, therefore, that the effect is probably due to an interaction of the ligand and regulatory site as opposed to a chemical
modification (phosphorylation) of one of the components of the
adenylyl-cyclase system.

Purine nucleoside triphosphates were shown to enhance stimulation of adenylyl cyclase also in fat-cell ghosts (Fig. 4), pancreatic β-cells (Fig. 5), human platelets (19), as well as several

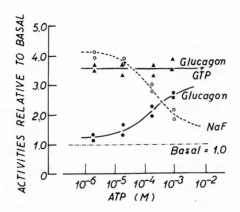

Fig. 5. Effect of ATP and GTP on response of adenylyl-cyclase
activity of pancreatic β cells to glucagon and fluoride. 1000 x g
particles prepared from insulin-secreting tumors of the Syrian
(golden) hamster (for details see Reference 104) were incubated in
0.06 ml for 2.5 minutes at $30°C$ with the indicated concentrations
of ATP in the presence of no addition (basal), 10 µg/ml glucagon,
10 µg/ml glucagon plus 10^{-5}M GTP and 10 mM NaF. Remaining incubation conditions were: 25 mM creatine phosphate, 1 mg/ml creatine
kinase, 0.33% albumin (human), 5 mM $MgCl_2$, and 50 mM Tris HCl
(pH 7.8). At each ATP concentration the stimulation of cyclic-AMP
production was expressed relative to that obtained under basal conditions. (From Ref. 13.)

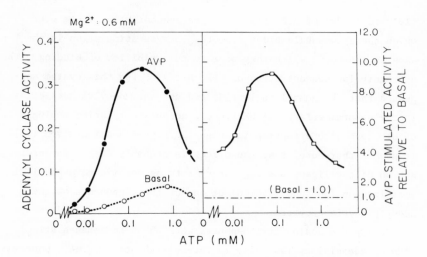

Fig. 6. Effect of ATP concentration on stimulation of beef renal medullary adenylyl-cyclase activity by 10^{-7}M AVP. AVP-stimulated activity relative to basal was calculated by dividing the activity obtained in the presence of AVP at each ATP concentration by the respective activity obtained in the absence of AVP. Incubations were for 10 minutes. Remaining conditions were same as those for Figure 2. Adenylyl-cyclase activities are expressed as nM cyclic AMP formed per mg protein per 10 minutes. (From Ref. 48.)

other systems. One of these, the neurohypophyseal-hormone(NHH)-sensitive adenylyl cyclase in membranes of beef renal medulla illustrates the complexity of this mode of regulation of stimulation.

As illustrated in Figure 6, ATP has both stimulatory and inhibitory effects on AVP response. The stimulatory effect is seen between 5 and 90 μM ATP; the inhibitory effect becomes evident when the concentration of ATP is increased further to 1.0 mM. Addition of GTP results in inhibition of AVP-stimulated activity without affecting basal activity. Concentrations of GTP as low as 5 x 10^{-8}M clearly affect this system; half-maximal inhibition is obtained with about 2 x 10^{-7}M (Fig. 7). Thus, the GTP-dependent step discovered in the glucagon-sensitive adenylyl-cyclase system in liver-plasma membranes does not seem to be an invariant feature of hormone-sensitive adenylyl-cyclase systems. This conclusion is supported by the findings of Wolff and Cook (21), who determined

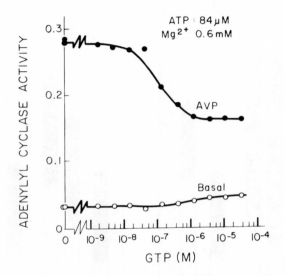

Fig. 7.   Effect of GTP on basal and AVP-stimulated adenylyl-cyclase activities in beef renal medullary membranes.   Renal medullary membranes were incubated in the presence of 84 μM ATP and 0.6 mM Mg^{2+} (in excess over 1.4 mM EDTA), and the indicated concentrations of GTP.   AVP when present was 10^{-7}M.   Remaining incubation conditions were same as those for Figure 2.   Adenylyl-cyclase activities are expressed as nM cyclic AMP formed per mg protein per 10 minutes.   (From Ref. 48.)

that the TSH response in beef thyroid membranes is preferentially stimulated by ITP rather than GTP, although the latter was also active.

Beef renal medullary membranes also contain a prostaglandin(PG)-sensitive adenylyl-cyclase system that is distinct from the AVP-sensitive system; changes in activities due to saturating concentrations of AVP and PG are additive.   In contrast to AVP, the effect of PGE_1 is dependent on the addition of micromolar concentrations of GTP or millimolar concentrations of ATP.   Figure 8 illustrates both effects of GTP; that inhibiting AVP response and that stimulating PGE_1 response.   It also shows that the effects of ATP and GTP on either adenylyl-cyclase system are not additive, suggesting that ATP, at concentrations approaching 1.0 mM, mimics the actions of GTP on both renal medullary adenylyl cyclases.

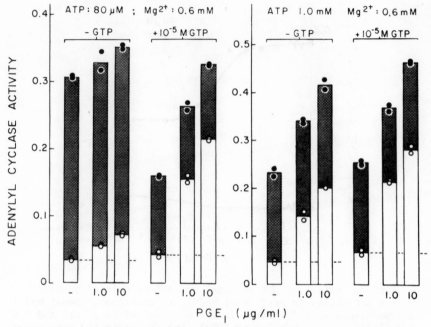

Fig. 8. Effect of GTP and ATP on stimulation of renal medullary adenylyl cyclase by PGE₁ and AVP. Beef renal medullary membranes (37/41.5% sucrose interface) were incubated for 10 minutes at 37°C with the indicated concentrations of ATP, MG^{2+} (excess over 1.4 mM EDTA), GTP, and prostaglandin E₁. Remaining incubation conditions were same as those for Figure 2. Open bars represent adenylyl-cyclase activity determined in the absence of AVP; hatched bars represent change in activity due to addition of 10^{-7}M AVP. Adenylyl-cyclase activities are expressed as nM cyclic AMP formed per mg protein per 10 minutes. (From Ref. 48.)

The characteristics of the stimulatory effect of ATP on AVP response seen between 5 and 90 μM ATP were also investigated. It was found that this effect is not specific for ATP. Adenosine and AMP, but not cyclic AMP, cyclic GMP, GMP, or cyclic IMP, mimic the effect of ATP in maximally stimulating the response of the renal system to AVP. The effects of adenosine and AMP at 3 x 10^{-5}M on the AVP-stimulated activity determined at 5 M ATP are shown in Figure 9. It was also found that the stimulatory effects of ATP and adenosine are not additive (Fig. 10), suggesting that these compounds act at the same site or through the same process. Neither

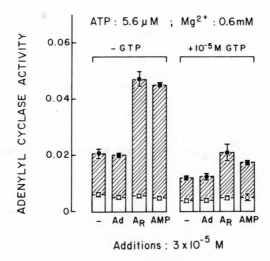

Additions : 3×10^{-5} M

Fig. 9.   Effect of adenine, adenosine, and AMP on basal and
AVP-stimulated adenylyl-cyclase activities in beef renal medullary
plasma membranes.   Renal medullary membranes (37/41.5% sucrose
interface) were incubated for 10 minutes at 37°C at the indicated
concentrations of ATP, Mg^{2+} (excess over 1.4 mM EDTA), GTP, adenine, adenosine, and AMP.   Open bars represent activities determined in the absence of AVP and hatched bars represent the change
in activity due to addition of 10^{-7}M AVP.   Remaining incubation
conditions were same as those for Figure 2.   Adenylyl-cyclase activities are expressed as nM cyclic AMP formed per mg protein per
10 minutes.   (From Ref. 48.)

adenosine (Fig. 10) nor AMP (not shown) interfere with the inhibi-

tory effect of GTP on AVP stimulation of adenylyl cyclase, suggest-

ing that adenosine or AMP act at sites different from those of GTP.

The stimulation of hormone action by adenosine and AMP is remi-

niscent of effects seen by Sattin and Rall (45) in brain slices.

These purine derivations led to increased cyclic-AMP levels and

potentiated the stimulatory action of histamine.   It will be inter-

esting to determine whether these two phenomena are related from a

mechanistic point of view.   Effects of nucleotides and nucleosides

were analyzed by expressing hormonal stimulation relative to basal

activity.   This mode of analysis corrects for any effect the

tested compound may have on basal activity, i.e., on the functional

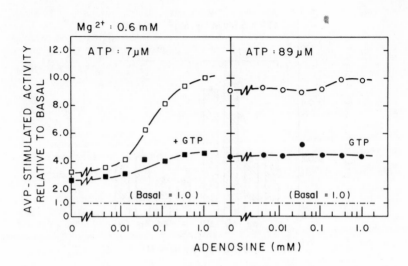

Fig. 10. Effect of varying concentrations of adenosine on hormonal stimulation of renal medullary membrane adenylyl-cyclase activity determined at suboptimal and optimal ATP concentrations. Incubations were for 10 minutes at 37°C. When present, GTP was 10^{-5}M and AVP, 10^{-7}M. Remaining incubation conditions were same as those for Figure 2. (From Ref. 48.)

state of the catalytic unit of the system. Depending on the system studied, purine derivatives (GTP, adenosine, AMP, and ITP) may have profound effects on the catalytic unit of the system, with or without affecting the susceptibility of the system to hormones. An example of this was recently reported by Fain et al. (46), who found that adenine nucleosides, particularly 2-deoxy-adenosine, at concentrations above 0.1 mM inhibit fat-cell adenylyl-cyclase activity without affecting the ratio between the remaining basal and hormonally stimulated activities. Studies by Leray et al. (20), on the other hand, demonstrated that in liver of adrenalectomized rats, addition of GTP results in increase of both epinephrine stimulation and basal activity. Fortuitously, GTP exerts only a small action on basal activity of the renal medullary membrane adenylyl cyclase and this facilitates analysis and interpretation; but this is not so with adenosine. At 0.5 mM, for example, this nucleoside both enhanced the relative AVP stimulation and inhibited

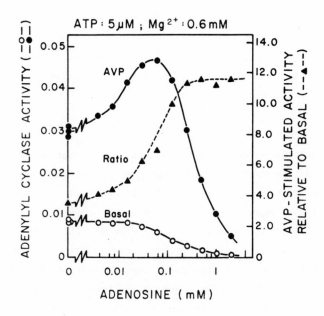

Fig. 11. Effect of varying concentrations of adenosine on adenylyl-cyclase activity determined in the absence and the presence of 10^{-7}M AVP. Concentrations of ATP and Mg^{2+} (excess over EDTA) were those indicated on the figure. Incubations were for 10 minutes at 37°C. Remaining incubation conditions were same as those for Figure 2. Adenylyl-cyclase activities are expressed as nM cyclic AMP formed per mg protein per 10 minutes. (From Ref. 48.)

the catalytic process (Fig. 11). Final interpretation of effects of nucleosides and nucleotides will have to take these "side-effects" into account.

In conclusion, experiments with beef renal medullary membranes suggest that ATP can interact with three distinct sites of the AVP-sensitive adenylyl-cyclase system: (1) catalytic sites, serving as a substrate, (2) regulatory site I, enhancing AVP response (this effect appears to be mimicked by adenosine and AMP), and (3) regulatory site II, inhibiting AVP response (mimicking the inhibitory effect of GTP). Like the existence of an allosteric site for Mg^{2+} in other adenylyl-cyclase systems (49), the actual existence of multiple regulatory sites in the AVP-sensitive adenylyl-cyclase

system is still a matter of speculation. The lesson to be learned
from these studies, however, is that nucleotides and nucleosides,
up to now purine derivatives, regulate the expression of hormonal
stimulation by acting, either as positive or negative modulators,
depending on the system studied.

FINAL REMARKS

It should be evident that considerable information has been
accumulated in recent years concerning the molecular nature and
function of hormone receptors coupled to adenylyl cyclases. Probing
the kinetics of adenylyl-cyclase activation has provided new insight
into the mode of action of hormones. However, the kinetics of the
hormonally induced activation process, the coupling of receptor to
adenylyl cyclase and the structural organization of the adenylyl-
cyclase system in the plasma membrane are basic problems still
unresolved. Hormone receptors and adenylyl cyclases may be organized in clusters across the membrane surface, which might account
for the complex non-Michaelian kinetics. The mode of coupling of
the hormone receptors and the adenylyl cyclases is an enigma. Two
possibilities come to mind: 1) either the receptor and the catalytic unit are permanently coupled, or 2) hormone receptors "float"
within the membrane, independent of the catalytic unit. In the
latter case, coupling and concomitant stimulation of activity is
established only while hormone binding to receptors takes place.
Temporary coupling of the hormone receptor with the catalytic unit
could be the basis for time delays and bursts of activity which are
observed in some of the adenylyl-cyclase systems studied. We hope
that molecular entities of these complex systems will soon be
isolated and provide insight into their structure and interactions.

ACKNOWLEDGMENTS

I should like to thank Drs. T. Braun and S. Sepsenwol of the
Department of Physiology, Northwestern University Medical School,
for critical review of this manuscript.

This research was supported in part by USPHS Grants No. HD-06513 and HD-06273.

REFERENCES

1. L. L. Miller, Recent Progr. Horm. Res., 17: 539 (1961).

2. J. H. Exton and C. R. Park, Advan. Enzyme Regul., 6: 391 (1968).

3. J. H. Exton and C. R. Park, J. Biol. Chem., 243: 4189 (1968).

4. F. A. Robinson, J. H. Exton, C. R. Park, and E. W. Sutherland, Fed. Proc. Fed. Amer. Soc. Exp. Biol., 26: 257 (1967).

5. J. H. Exton, G. A. Robinson, E. W. Sutherland, and C. R. Park, J. Biol. Chem., 246: 6167 (1971).

6. T. F. Williams, J. H. Exton, N. Friedmann, and C. R. Park, Amer. J. Physiol., 221: 1645 (1971).

7. V. Mutt and J. W. Jorpes, Recent Progr. Horm. Res., 23: 483 (1967).

8. P. W. Feltx, M. E. C. Ferguson, K. A. Hagey, E. S. Stitt, and W. M. Mitchell, Diabetalogia, 6: 44 (1970).

9. F. Sundby, Excerpta Medica ICS, 209: 80 (1970).

10. S. L. Pohl, L. Birnbaumer, M. Rodbell, J. Biol. Chem., 246: 1849 (1971).

11. M. Rodbell, L. Birnbaumer, S. L. Pohl, and F. Sundby, Proc. Nat. Acad. Sci. USA, 68: 909 (1971).

12. M. Rodbell, M. Lin, and Y. Solomon, J. Biol. Chem., 249: 59 (1974).

13. I. D. Goldfine, J. Roth, and L. Birnbaumer, J. Biol. Chem., 247: 1211 (1972).

14. F. Murad and M. Vaughan, Biochem. Pharmacol., 18: 1053 (1969).

15. G. A. Robison, R. W. Butcher, and E. W. Sutherland, Ann. N.Y. Acad. Sci., 139: 703 (1967).

16. R. W. Butcher, C. E. Baird, and E. W. Sutherland, J. Biol. Chem., 243: 1705 (1968).

17. L. Birnbaumer and M. Rodbell, J. Biol. Chem., 244: 3477 (1969).

18. M. Rodbell, L. Birnbaumer, S. L. Pohl, and H. M. J. Krans, J. Biol. Chem., 246: 1877 (1971).

19. G. Krishna, J. Harwood, A. J. Barber, and G. A. Jamieson, J. Biol. Chem., 247: 2253 (1972).

20. F. Leray, A. M. Chambaut and J. Janoune, Biochem. Biophys. Res. Comm., 48: 1385 (1972).

21. J. Wolf and G. H. Cook, J. Biol. Chem., 248: 350 (1973).

22. M. Rodbell, H. M. J. Krans, S. L. Pohl, and L. Birnbaumer, J. Biol. Chem., 247: 1861 (1971).

23. P. Cuatrecasas, Proc. Nat. Acad. Sci. U.S., 68: 1264 (1971).

24. B. J. Campbell, G. Woodward, and B. Borberg, J. Biol. Chem., 247: 6167 (1972).

25. R. J. Lefkowitz, G. W. G. Sharp, and E. Haber, J. Biol. Chem., 248: 342 (1973).

26. C. Y. Lee and R. J. Ryan, Biochemistry, 12: 4609 (1973).

27. J. Bockaert, Ch. Roy, R. Rayerison, and S. Jard, J. Biol. Chem., 248: 5923 (1973).

28. L. Birnbaumer, S. L. Pohl, M. Rodbell, and F. Sundby, J. Biol. Chem., 247: 2038 (1972).

29. L. Birnbaumer, Excerpta Medica ICS, 241: 471 (1972).

30. S. L. Pohl, H. M. J. Krans, L. Birnbaumer, and M. Rodbell, J. Biol. Chem., 247: 2295 (1972).

31. M. Rodbell, A. B. Jones, G. E. Chiappe de Cingolani, and L. Birnbaumer, Recent Progr. Horm. Res., 24: 215 (1968).

32. M. W. Bitensky, R. E. Gorman, A. H. Neufeld, and R. King, Endocrinology, 89: 1242 (1971).

33. M. Rodbell, H. M. J. Krans, S. L. Pohl, and L. Birnbaumer, J. Biol. Chem., 246: 1872 (1971).

34. S. L. Pohl, H. M. J. Krans, V. Kozyreff, L. Birnbaumer, and M. Rodbell, J. Biol. Chem., 246: 4447 (1971).

35. L. Birnbaumer and S. L. Pohl, J. Biol. Chem., 248: 2056 (1973).

36. F. Murad, B. S. Strauch, and M. Vaughan, Biochem. Biophys. Acta, 177: 591 (1969).

37. J. P. Harwood, H. Low, and M. Rodbell, J. Biol. Chem., 248: 6239 (1973).

38. C. Frieden, J. Biol. Chem., 245: 5788 (1970).

39. G. R. Ainslie, Jr., J. P. Shill, and K. E. Neet, J. Biol. Chem., 247: 7088 (1972).

40. L. Birnbaumer, S. L. Pohl, and M. Rodbell, Advanc. Biochem. Psychopharmacol., 3: 185 (1970).

41. G. S. Levey, Ann. N.Y. Acad. Sci., 185: 449 (1971).

42. G. S. Levey, Biochem. Biophys. Res. Comm., 42: 103 (1971).

43. G. S. Levey, J. Biol. Chem., 246: 7905 (1971).

44. R. G. Young, D. Babcock, W. Ballantyne, and D. Ojala,
     Biochemistry, 10: 2484 (1971).

45. A. Sattin and R. W. Rall, Mol. Pharmacol., 6: 13 (1970).

46. J. N. Fain, R. H. Pointer, and W. F. Ward, J. Biol. Chem.,
     247: 6866 (1972).

47. G. Krishna, B. Weiss, and B. B. Brodie, J. Pharm. Exp. Therap.,
     163: 379 (1968).

48. L. Birnbaumer, Biochim. Biophys. Acta, 300: 129 (1973).

49. L. Birnbaumer, S. L. Pohl, and M. Rodbell, J. Biol. Chem.,
     244: 3468 (1969).

Chapter 12

EFFECTS OF ADRENERGIC COMPOUNDS
ON THE ADENYLATE CYCLASE OF FROG ERYTHROCYTES

Carl Grunfeld
Department of Pharmacology
Albert Einstein College of Medicine
Bronx, New York

Jack Erlichman
Department of Molecular Biology
Albert Einstein College of Medicine
Bronx, New York

Ora M. Rosen
Departments of Medicine and Molecular Biology
Albert Einstein College of Medicine
Bronx, New York

This review will summarize some of the biochemical features of the adenylate-cyclase systems of frog and tadpole erythrocytes, the acquisition of catecholamine sensitivity by the tadpole erythrocyte during metamorphosis, and the structure-activity relationships for some of the adrenergic agents which influence frog-erythrocyte adenylate cyclase.

Although mature mammalian erythrocytes contain little adenylate-cyclase activity, this activity is readily demonstrated in the nucleated erythrocytes of birds (1,2) and amphibia (3)*. The requirements for activity of the adenylate-cyclase system in frog and tadpole lysates are similar to those described for a variety of mammalian adenylate cyclases (3). Activity measured in the presence of NaF is dependent upon Mg^{2+} and shows a partial requirement for sulfhydryl-containing compounds and a phosphodiesterase inhi-

---

*Cyclic-AMP formation from radioactive ATP was assayed by a modification of the method of Weiss & Costa (4). Following the incubation, noncyclic nucleotides were precipitated by $BaSO_4$ and the cyclic AMP in the supernatant fluid was purified by paper chromatography (5).

bitor (theophylline). The specific activities of adenylate cyclase
in crude lysates from frog and tadpole erythrocytes (measured in
the presence of NaF) are 0.3 and 0.2 nM cyclic AMP formed per
minute/milligram protein respectively. In the absence of NaF,
catecholamines activate frog erythrocyte adenylate cyclase. Maximal activation occurs with 10^{-4}M isoproterenol and represents 50%
of the activity inducible by the addition of 0.01M NaF. The order
of potency is isoproterenol>epinephrine>norepinephrine. Essentially
no activity is seen in the absence of either NaF or catecholamines.
Activation by catecholamines is blocked by β-adrenergic blockers
but not by α-adrenergic blockers such as dibenzyline or phentolamine.

Activation by catecholamines occurs rapidly (< 2 minutes) and
proceeds linearly for about 10 to 15 min. Many other hormones
tested exhibited no activity in either the presence or absence of
catecholamines, e.g., insulin, glucagon, ACTH, vasopressin, thyroxine, and triiodothyronine, as well as prostaglandins and serotonin.
Thus the hormonal sensitivity of this adenylate-cyclase system
appears to be simple and similar to that expected for a β-adrenergic
receptor.

The adenylate cyclase of the tadpole erythrocyte, unlike that
of the frog, does not respond to either catecholamines or other
hormones, although it is nearly as active as the frog enzyme in the
presence of NaF. Lack of sensitivity to catecholamines is not a
result of the method used to lyse the cells or the concentration of
hormone added. Intact erythrocytes, incubated with [^{3}H]-adenosine,
rapidly convert it to [^{3}H]-ATP. If such cells are then washed and
incubated in the presence of methylxanthines, [^{3}H]-cyclic AMP
accumulates in both frog and tadpole erythrocytes, but only the
frog erythrocytes respond to the addition of exogenous catecholamines by increasing the amount of [^{3}H]-cyclic AMP formed (6).

In order to determine the onset of hormonal sensitivity by
tadpole-erythrocyte adenylate cyclase, premetamorphic tadpoles were
treated with gradually increasing concentrations of thyroxine in
order to induce metamorphosis in the laboratory (6). During development of hind legs and the emergence of front legs, there was no

evidence of sensitivity to catecholamines.   Only after tail shortening began did sensitivity appear and approach that seen in adult
frogs (upon completion of metamorphosis).   Tadpoles undergoing
natural metamorphosis, i.e., in the absence of exogenous thyroxine,
also followed this pattern.   Interestingly, the development of
catecholamine-sensitive adenylate cyclase paralleled the emergence of
frog hemoglobin, as detected by polyacrylamide-gel electrophoresis.

A fundamental, as yet unsettled question is whether there is one
population of erythrocytes, which, during the course of metamorphosis, acquires a hormone receptor that is integrated with the catalytic moiety of adenylate cyclase in such fashion as to yield a
hormone-sensitive enzyme system, or alternatively, whether there is
a new clone of adult frog erythrocytes arising at this time that
contains a different adenylate-cyclase system, sensitive to catecholamines.   Another possibility is that the hormone receptor is
present throughout development and only becomes integrated with the
adenylate-cyclase system during development.   An attempt to dif-
ferentiate these alternatives by studying the binding of $[^3H]$-
epinephrine to frog- and tadpole-erythrocyte membranes is in progress.

The membrane-bound adenylate cyclases of both frog and tadpole
erythrocytes were partially purified (7).   The enzyme from frog
erythrocytes retained its sensitivity to activation by either NaF
or catecholamines, whereas that from the tadpole erythrocytes re-
mained insensitive to the addition of catecholamines.   These
preparations of adenylate cyclase did not contain cyclic nucleotide
phosphodiesterase but required the addition of sulfhydryl-containing
compounds for activity.

Since the purified frog adenylate cyclase exhibited the properties of a β-adrenergic receptor, we decided to test a variety of
adrenergic agents in order to more precisely define the chemical
events occurring during hormone stimulation and blockade and the
relationship between activity in the enzyme assay and that observed
in intact-organ and whole-animal preparations.   In an initial study
(8), we found that compounds lacking a hydroxyl at the β-carbon
failed to stimulate adenylate-cyclase activity or to block stimu-

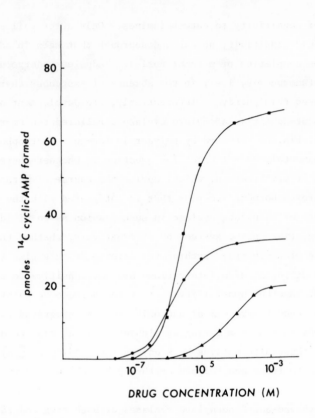

DRUG CONCENTRATION (M)

FIG. 1. Activation of adenylate cyclase by β-adrenergic
agonists. Enzyme [10μg, (8)] was incubated for 15 minutes at 37°
in the presence of 50 mM Tris-HCl buffer, pH 8.1; 3 mM MgSO₄, 20 mM
dithiothreitol; 1 mM [14C]-ATP (1000 cpm/nmole); and drug. Isoproterenol (■), Soterenol (●), β-desoxysoterenol (▲). (From
Ref. 9.)

lation by catecholamines. Dopamine, tyramine, hydroxyamphetamine,

methoxyphenamine and other compounds tested do not, however, have

the large amine substitution that is important for β-adrenergic

activity. Some of these also do not fulfill the requirements we

eventually established for substitutions on the ring. β-deoxyso-

terenol and β-desoxyisoproterenol, which have N-isopropyl groups,

did stimulate cyclase activity (9). In Figure 1, stimulation by

soterenol, its β-desoxy congener and isoproterenol are compared.

Absence of a β hydroxyl drastically reduces the affinity as well as

the intrinsic activity of a drug. (The d-isomer of soterenol is

also a weak activator). Trimethoquinol, a tetrahydroisoquinoline
with pharmacological activity as a bronchodilator, has been viewed
as a β-desoxy analogue of the catecholamines (10). It weakly stimulates adenylate cyclase, but, unlike other β-desoxy compounds, has
a high apparent affinity. We can conclude from a study of these
drugs that a β-hydroxyl group is not absolutely required for agonist
activity.

Compounds with two hydroxyls on the ring, like the catecholamines, stimulate adenylate-cyclase activity, whereas drugs with
one hydroxyl, whether in the 4 position as in nylidrin or in the
3 position as in S 40045-9, do not (Table 1). Compounds containing
single hydroxyls have been reported to have significant β-adrenergic
activity in vivo (11). These drugs do bind to the receptor since,
as we will show later, they are potent inhibitors of catecholamine-
stimulated adenylate cyclase. Two functional groups appear to be
required for stimulation of adenylate-cyclase activity in vivo.

It is possible to substitute certain functional groups other
than hydroxyls in the 3 position and still retain activity. Two
β_2 agonists, soterenol, with a methanesulfonamide, and salbutamol,
with a hydroxymethyl in the 3 position, stimulate the enzyme, but to
a smaller degree than isoproterenol. These functional groups share
the property of being able to donate a proton in a hydrogen bond,
which may account for both the inactivity of MJ 9646, a drug in
which the amide has been substituted with a methyl group, and the
inactivity in vivo of 3-methoxy metabolites of catecholamines.

If the groups on the rings are reversed, as in an isomer of
soterenol, with the bulky methanesulfonamide group in the 4 position,
the drug does not stimulate even though the substituent in the

3 position is able to donate a proton. Both the reversed isomer
of soterenol and the similar analogue of salbutamol are inactive in
intact organ preparations (12).

A hydroxyl at the 4 position is not an absolute requirement
since metaproterenol possesses two metahydroxyls and is a weak
agonist (see Table 1). Larsen (13) has proposed a quinone-methide
transition as a mechanism for β-adrenergic stimulation. Metaproterenol, however, does not have a 4-hydroxyl and therefore cannot

TABLE 1

RING SUBSTITUTIONS [a]

STIMULATE	DO NOT STIMULATE
ISOPROTERENOL (100%)	NYLIDRIN
$HO-C_6H_3(HO)-CHCH_2NHCH(CH_3)_2$, OH	$HO-C_6H_4-CHCH_2NH\overset{CH_3}{\underset{CH_2CH_2\phi}{C}H}$, OH
SOTERENOL (50%)	S 40045-9
$HO-C_6H_3(CH_3SO_2NH)-CHCH_2NHCH(CH_3)_2$, OH	$HO-C_6H_4-CHCH_2NHCH(CH_3)_2$, OH
SALBUTAMOL (65%)	REVERSE SOTERENOL
$HO-C_6H_3(HOCH_2)-CHCH_2NHCH(CH_3)_2$, OH	$CH_3SO_2NH-C_6H_3(HO)-CHCH_2NHCH(CH_3)_2$, OH
METAPROTERENOL (25%)	MJ 9646
$HO-C_6H_3(HO)-CHCH_2NHCH(CH_3)_2$, OH	$HO-C_6H_3(CH_3SO_2N(CH_3))-CHCH_2NHCH(CH_3)_2$, OH
MJ 9910 (13%)	
$HO-C_6H_3(HO)-OCH_2CHCH_2NHCH(CH_3)_2$, OH	
QUINTERENOL (40%)	
$HO-C_9H_5N-CHCH_2NHCH(CH_3)_2$, OH	
TRIMETHOQUINOL (17%)	
(tetrahydroisoquinoline) HO, HO ring; $CH_2-C_6H_2(OCH_3)_3$	

[a] The percentages in parentheses indicate the intrinsic activity of the compound relative to that of isoproterenol.

TABLE 2

INHIBITORS [a]

SOTALOL (1.0)	CH$_3$SO$_2$NH—⟨⟩—CHCH$_2$NHCH(CH$_3$) $\quad$ OH
METALOL (.35)	$\qquad$ CH$_3$ CH$_3$SO$_2$NH—⟨⟩—CHCHNHCH$_3$ $\quad$ OH
AMIDEPHRINE (.06)	⟨⟩—CHCHNHCH$_3$ CH$_3$SO$_2$NH $\quad$ OH
α–METHYLSOTALOL (1.0)	$\qquad$ CH$_3$ CH$_3$SO$_2$NH—⟨⟩—CHCHNHCH(CH$_3$)$_2$ $\quad$ OH
MJ 9646 (.92)	HO—⟨⟩—CHCH$_2$NHCH(CH$_3$)$_2$ CH$_3$SO$_2$N $\quad$ OH $\quad$ CH$_3$
REVERSE SOTERENOL (.02)	CH$_3$SO$_2$NH—⟨⟩—CHCH$_2$NHCH(CH$_3$)$_2$ HO $\quad$ OH
TRIMETHOQUINOL (20)	HO—⟨⟩ N ⟩—OCH$_3$ CH$_2$—⟨⟩—OCH$_3$ $\quad$ OCH$_3$
PROPRANOLOL (36)	⟨⟩—OCH$_2$CHCH$_2$NHCH(CH$_3$)$_2$ $\quad$ OH

[a] The numbers in parentheses indicate the potency of the inhibitors relative to sotalol which is taken as 1.0

undergo this reaction. Another agonist, the aryloxypropanolamine,
MJ-9910, is also unable to make such a transition because of the
oxygen bridge between the phenyl ring and the propanolamine side
chain.

Quinterenol, an agonist, is a 5-substituted 8-hydroxyquinoline.
If the 8-hydroxyl group is equated with the 4 position of catecholamines, then the aromatic nitrogen may be in the equivalent of the
3 position. Unlike the 3 substituents of the other agonists, the
aromatic amine cannot donate a hydrogen. This assumption of equi-
valence, however, may not be correct because, unlike the rings of
the other agonists, the quinoline ring system of quinterenol does
not have free rotation with respect to the ethanolamine side chain.

β-adrenergic blocking activity was tested by incubating adenylate cyclase in the presence of isoproterenol (5×10^{-5}M) and varying concentrations of adrenergic blockers (see Table 2). Racemic
sotalol and dichloroisoproterenol are equipotent in blocking the
stimulation by isoproterenol. Nylidrin, the monohydroxy compound
mentioned earlier, and propranolol, are more potent. l-Sotalol was
2½ times as potent and d-sotalol 6/100 as potent as the racemic
drug.

Metalol, an N-methyl analogue of sotalol is 1/3 as potent as
sotalol. Amidephrine, with a methanesulfonamide in the 3 position
and a methyl-substituted amine, is 1/17 as potent as sotalol or
approximately 1/6 as potent as the 4-substituted metalol. The equivalent potency of α-methyl cogeners, demonstrated here with sotalol,
enable us to compare metalol and amidephrine although one lacks an
α-methyl substitution. Thus, with a single ring substitution, a
methanesulfonamide in the 4 position gives a more active blocker
than when it is present in the 3 position.

Blocking characteristics are changed if a second functional
group, a hydroxyl, is added. MJ 9646, the sulfonamide N-methyl-
substituted analogue of soterenol, is as potent a blocker as sotalol.
It has a sulfonamide in the 3 position and a hydroxyl in the
4 position. The reversed analogue of soterenol with a 4-sulfonamide
and a 3-hydroxyl is a poorer blocker. This may be due to the re-

TABLE 3

Effect of Blockers on Activation of Adenylate Cyclase[a]

Activator	Blocker	Activity pM cAMP formed per minute	%
Epinephrine	None	18.7	100
	S 38537-9	15.9	85
	Dichloroisoproterenol	3.9	21
	Buphenine	3.4	18
Ethylnorepinephrine	None	23.5	100
	S 38537-9	21.3	91
	Dichloroisoproterenol	6.7	28
	Buphenine	3.8	16
Isoproterenol	None	24.6	100
	S 38537-9	23.2	98
	Dichloroisoproterenol	11.3	46
	Buphenine	7.9	32
AH3923	None	11.3	100
	S 38537-9	13.1	116
	Dichloroisoproterenol	9.4	83
	Buphenine	5.1	45
Prokokylol	None	25.2	100
	S 38537-9	24.6	98
	Dichloroisoproterenol	21.2	84
	Buphenine	11.9	47

[a]The final concentration of activators and blockers was
  $5 \times 10^{-5}M$.   (8)

stricted rotation of the 4-sulfonamide in the presence of a
3-hydroxyl.

The role of the amine substituent in blockade is demonstrated
in Table 3. The size of the amine substitution increases from drug
S 38,537 to nylidrin. Blockers with large N substituents are better
able to block activation induced by agonists with large N substituents. Finally, with regard to blockers, drugs like trimethoquinol
with low activity but high apparent affinity, can function in this
assay as antagonists to the more active isoproterenol. Inhibition
by trimethoquinol never exceeds 80%, however, due to its own intrinsic activity.

Many authors have proposed chemical mechanisms for the adrenergic receptor based on structure-activity studies performed in intact organs and whole animals (14). The effects of drugs, in such preparations, are dependent upon route of administration, metabolism, and interaction with nonadrenergic receptors mediating similar physiological responses. In addition, adrenergic agents may produce an "indirect" sympathomimetic effect. The proposal by Robison, Butcher, and Sutherland (15) that β receptors may be regulatory subunits of adenylate cyclase suggests that direct studies of this enzyme system might yield information independent of the complications observed with studies performed in vivo. Thus we have collected structure-activity data using an adenylate-cyclase preparation which appears to contain a β-adrenergic receptor site in order to assess the requirements for activation.

In addition to the general characteristics of β stimulation, i.e., greater responsiveness to drugs with large amine substitutions, and blockade by β rather than α blockers, this enzyme possesses the SAR characteristics of the β_2 receptor responsible for bronchodilation and vasodilation (16). The α-methyl substitutions do not decrease the activity of agonists such as cobefrine (which is α-methyl norepinephrine) (8), or of antagonists such as α-methyl sotalol. Three predominantly bronchodilating drugs, salbutamol, quinterenol, and trimethoquinol, effectively stimulate adenylate-cyclase activity. Adenylate-cyclase preparations from heart and lung have, in fact, been shown to reflect the hormone responsiveness of the β_1 and β_2 receptors, respectively (17).

While our structure-activity study allows us to identify frog-erythrocyte adenylate cyclase as a model β_2 receptor, the number of drugs tested does not permit us to draw definitive conclusions as to the chemical mechanism involved in adrenergic stimulation. Several general principles may be formulated, however, about the role of various substitutions in interactions with the receptor. The ring substitutions show structural specificity with regard to stimulation, and contribute more to the intrinsic activity than the affinity of most drugs. The amine substitution contributes to both intrinsic activity and affinity (8). The role of the β-hydroxyl group is less clear but it often contributes more to the affinity than to the intrinsic activity.

Whereas direct drug-receptor interactions are easier to study in our in vitro assay, it is difficult to correlate the potency of drugs in this kind of assay with the potency of the adrenergic response in whole animals and tissue preparations, since the amount of cyclic AMP formed after adenylate-cyclase stimulation in vitro may exceed the level necessary to induce a β-adrenergic response (18). Two values, apparent affinity and intrinsic activity are needed to characterize enzyme stimulation. Since excess cyclic AMP may be formed in response to the addition of hormones or drugs, measurement of apparent affinity may be more relevant to the psychological adrenergic response. Thus, the ability of drugs like

TABLE 4

Comparative Effects of Adrenergic Agonists and Antagonists on Frog Erythrocyte Adenylate Cyclase and on Tissue Preparations Reported in the Literature[a]

	Agonism		Blockade	
Compound	Adenylate Cyclase	Tissue Preparations	Adenylate Cyclase	Tissue Preparations
Isoproterenol	+++	+++		
Epinephrine	++	++		
Norepinephrine	++	+		
Dopamine	0	+,0		
Phenisonone	0	+		
Nylidrin	0	+,0	++	
Isoxsuprine	0	+,0	++	
S 40045-9	0	+	+	
Soterenol	+++	+++		
Salbutamol	++	++		
Trimethoquinol	+++	++	++	
Metaproterenol	+	+		
Quinterenol	++	++		
MJ-9910	+++	++		
Sotalol	0		++	++
Metalol	0		+	+
Amidephrine	0		±	±
Dichloroisopro- terenol	0		++	++

[a]For more complete compilation including references see Ref. 21.

130   C. GRUNFELD, J. ERLICHMAN, AND O. M. ROSEN

soterenol, quinterenol, and trimethoquinol to give a maximal adrenergic response is not inconsistent with their submaximal intrinsic
activity in the adenylate-cyclase assay.

The apparent affinities of many of the adrenergic drugs we
have tested are compared in Table 4, along with published results
on the effect of these drugs in tissue preparations. There is good
correlation between the two approaches, with two exceptions:
1) Dopamine and its analogues, which do not stimulate this adenylate-cyclase preparation are active in vivo, although the magnitude
of their direct adrenergic effect is open to question (19).
β-hydroxylation of dopamine leading to the formation of norepinephrine may occur in vivo. 2) The monohydroxylated ring compounds,
like nylidrin and isoxsuprine, which are also inactive in our assay,
have been classified as β-adrenergic agents (11). Their induction
of vasodilation, however, is not inhibited by β blockers and their
effect on uterine relaxation is only inhibited by β blockers in
vivo. In addition, they are known to act by several alternative
mechanisms and may be oxidized to catechols (20).

In conclusion, the adenylate cyclase of the amphibian erythrocyte offers advantages for the study of a β-adrenergic receptor
during development. The structural requirements for affinity and
intrinsic activity of adrenergic drugs with respect to adenylate-
cyclase activity can be analyzed. Further studies on drug-binding
to the receptor and correlation of this with the structure-activity
relationships for adenylate cyclase stimulation may lead to the
elucidation of a chemical mechanism of action for adrenergic agents.
Finally, quantitation of the relationship between cyclic-AMP
formation and physiological reactions will increase our understanding of the molecular basis of the adrenergic response.

ACKNOWLEDGMENT

These investigations were supported by USPHS, NIH Grants 5T5
GM 1674, AM 09033, and CA 10666 and American Cancer Society Grant
BC-12B. This paper was Communication No. 300 from the Joan and
Lester Avnet Institute of Molecular Biology.

REFERENCES

1. I. Oye and E. W. Sutherland, Biochim. Biophys. Acta, 127: 347 (1966).

2. P. R. Davoren and E. W. Sutherland, J. Biol. Chem., 238: 3009 (1963).

3. O. M. Rosen and S. M. Rosen, Biochem. Biophys. Res. Comm., 31: 82 (1968).

4. B. Weiss and E. Costa, Science, 156: 1750 (1967).

5. M. Hirata and O. Hayashi, Biochim. Biophys. Acta, 149: 1 (1967).

6. O. M. Rosen and J. Erlichman, Arch. Biochem. Biophys., 133: 171 (1969).

7. O. M. Rosen and S. M. Rosen, Arch. Biochem. Biophys., 131: 449 (1969).

8. O. M. Rosen, J. Erlichman, and S. M. Rosen, Mol. Pharm., 6: 524 (1970).

9. C. Grunfeld and O. M. Rosen, The Pharmacologist, 13: 256 (1970).

10. Y. Iwasawa and A. Kiyomoto, Jap. J. Pharmacol., 17: 143 (1967).

11. L. S. Goodman and A. Gilman, "The pharmacological basis of therapeutics", MacMillan, N.Y., 1971, p. 561.

12. A. A. Larsen, W. A. Gould, W. T. Comer, R. H. Uloth, K. W. Dungan, and P. M. Lish, J. Med. Chem., 10: 462 (1967); D. Hartley, D. Jack., L. H. C. Lunts, and A. C. Ritchie, Nature (London), 219: 861 (1968).

13. A. A. Larsen, Nature (London), 224: 25 (1969).

14. B. Belleau, Ann. N.Y. Acad. Sci., 139: 580 (1967); B. M. Bloom and I. M. Goldman, Adv. Drug Res., 3: 121 (1966).

15. G. A. Robison, R. W. Butcher, and E. W. Sutherland, in "Fundamental concepts in drug receptor interactions," eds. J. F. Danielli, N. F. Moran, and D. F. Triggle, Academic Press, N.Y., 1970, pp. 59-91.

16. A. M. Lands, A. Arnold, J. P. McAulift, F. P. Luduena, and T. G. Brown, Nature (London), 214: 597 (1967); A. M. Lands and T. G. Brown, Proc. Soc. Exp. Biol. Med., 116: 331 (1964).

17. R. A. Burges and K. J. Blackburn, Nature (London), 235: 249 (1972).

18. V. C. Manganiello, F. Murad, and M. Vaughan, J. Biol. Chem., 246: 2195 (1971).

19. T. H. Tsai, S. Z. Langer, and U. Trendelenburg, J. Pharm. Exp. Therp., 156: 321 (1967).

20. E. S. Manley and J. W. Lawson, Arch. Int. Pharmacody, 175: 239 (1968); R. W. Stander, Amer. J. Obs. Gyn., 94: 749 (1966).

21. C. Grunfeld, A. P. Grollman, and O. M. Rosen, Mol. Pharm., 10: 605 (1974).

Chapter 13

CALCIUM AND SKELETAL MUSCLE

C. Paul Bianchi

Department of Pharmacology
University of Pennsylvania School of Medicine
Philadelphia, Pa.

The role of calcium with regard to its function as a control
system has already been touched upon. I think if we turn our
attention to the physiology of the system, we can see certain relationships that place calcium in a unique role to act as a trigger,
governing very rapid coupling steps in excitable tissues such as
muscles.

In a cell of frog sartorius muscle there is 100 mM sodium
outside and potassium is 1½ to 3 mM, depending on the Ringer solution. The calcium level outside is 10^{-3} M. Inside the cell is a
store of approximately 1½ to 2 µM/g of calcium. The magnesium
level is on the order of 8 to 10 µM/g, of which about 3 µM may be
considered, by our best estimate, as being free.

Most enzyme systems are activated by magnesium and require
magnesium as a cofactor. In many instances calcium is indeed an
inhibitor of intracellular events or enzyme systems, except in some
very specific conditions in which the enzyme or the binding site,
to act as an activator for a sequence, requires calcium at very low
levels. I will discuss two coupling systems. In the first, the
calcium requirement for activation of contraction is approximately
10^{-7}M to 10^{-6}M—the range in which muscle goes from a relaxed state
to a maximally contracted state. The second coupling system also

requires calcium, but not specifically; that is, the function of
calcium may be performed by nickel or other divalent ions (except
magnesium). The requirement for calcium at this site is between
10^{-9} M and 10^{-7} M. This system is activated by calcium levels
below that at which contraction occurs, and, in addition, we believe that it requires cyclic AMP.

In skeletal muscle there is an electrical event, or action potential, on the order of 5 milliseconds which leads to a triggered
contractile response of the muscle lasting about 100 milliseconds
(Fig. 1). Essentially, this states the problem confronting us:
How can an electrical event of such short duration lead to a contractile response which is reversible, that is, in which there is
contraction and relaxation, and whose length of time is about 100
milliseconds?

The current hypothesis is that the action potential is propa-
gated down the transverse tubular element (1) and that there is a
coupling step between the transverse tubular elements and the terminal cisterni, which are the storage and release sites for calcium.
Functional disruption of the terminal cisternae by, say, batra-
choloxin (2), or the disruption of the transverse tubular element
by glycerol treatment (3) will interfere with the coupling step.
The trigger step is associated with a calcium requirement. The
exact nature of this requirement is not known. It may be that calcium is released from the transverse tubular element, acting as a
seeding event altering the membrane of the terminal cisternae and
thus causing a release of a quantity of calcium sufficient to bind
to the troponin sites. The longitudinal reticulum of the skeletal
muscle fiber is pictured as the site at which calcium is reaccumu-
lated at a slower rate and restored to the terminal cisternae. An
action potential, or the raising of the external potassium level
can trigger this step, in which case there is a depolarization and
phasic contraction of skeletal muscle. That is, contraction is a
self-limiting process when it's triggered by a depolarizing event
occurring at the membrane. This system in skeletal muscle is very

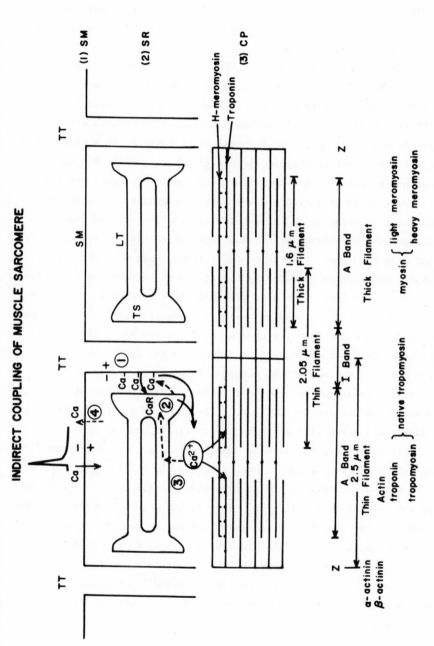

FIG. 1. Indirect coupling of muscle sarcomere.

resistant to removal of external calcium. It takes hours to deplete
the muscle tissue of calcium, and the cycle that is presented is essentially an internal one.

Two agents, potassium and caffeine, are primarily used to produce either excitation-respiration coupling (the increase of oxygen
uptake produced by raising external potassium) or excitation-contraction coupling (the potassium depolarization induced during a
phasic contraction). The pharmacology of caffeine in skeletal muscle is such that at very low levels (1 mM or less) it has an effect
on the increase in calcium influx. No tension is developed unless
contraction is triggered, in which case potentiated contraction is
due to a lowering of the threshold for coupling between depolarization and the release of calcium from the terminal cisterna. If
one goes to higher caffeine concentrations, then what one sees is a
phasic contraction produced by the action of caffeine on the sarcoplasmic reticulum. Congruent with this is the release of calcium of
the terminal cisterni and an associated contraction. The difference
between these two coupling agents, caffeine and potassium, is that
with potassium, there is a requirement for calcium to be bound in
the external surface of the membrane in order to have coupling
between depolarization and the release of calcium; whereas caffeine,
even in the presence of EDTA, will release this store of calcium,
and by this means will activate events within the sarcoplasm.

If we use higher caffeine concentrations, then the system goes
to pot. Caffeine action becomes irreversible and is associated with
a sustained contracture and an inhibition of the uptake of calcium
by the sarcoplasmic reticulum. That is the sequence of events with
regard to the contractile process. Before one sees an effect of
caffeine on the contractile process, one observes a marked increase
in heat production and oxygen uptake. Therefore, caffeine has an
effect on the ability of the muscle to metabolize and take up oxygen at a concentration that does not have an effect on the contractile process.

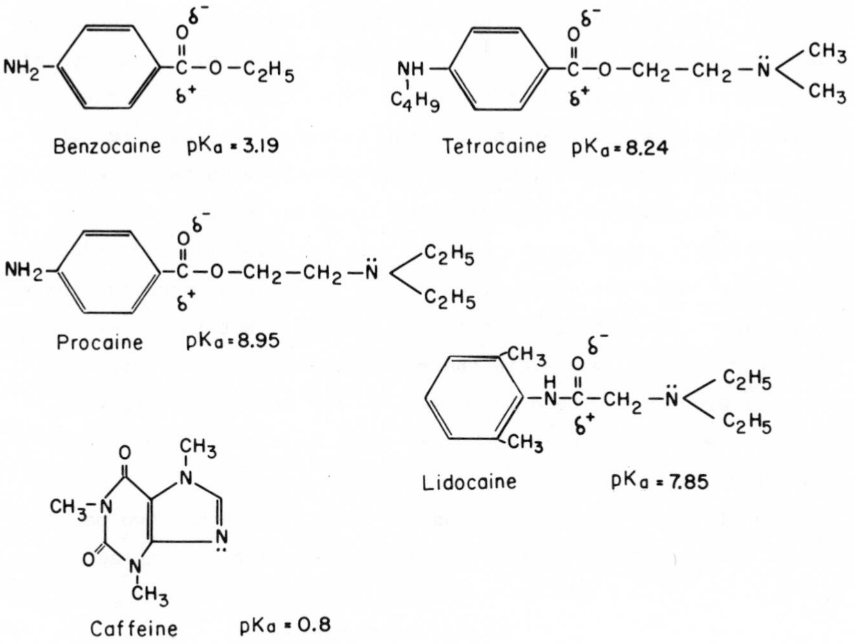

FIG. 2.   Association constants of local anesthetics and caffeine.

There is another group of agents which deserves mention at this point. Mostly they fall into two classes. The first is local anesthetics and the second is volatile anesthetics. In the case of the local anesthetics one has benzocaine, procaine, and tetracaine. (The association constants of these local anesthetics are given in Figure 2.) Tetracaine and procaine have the capability of competing with caffeine and blocking the caffeine-produced contraction. This is a function of the charged form of the local anesthetic. However, the major group involved in blocking caffeine contraction is not the charged tertiary amine moiety, but rather the carbonyl group (benzocaine quite effectively blocks the caffeine contracture). If the para amino group is transferred to the ortho position in benzocaine it is no longer capable of blocking the caffeine contracture; therefore it is the carbonyl group that we feel is

involved in competing with the caffeine for some site on the sarcoplasmic reticulum and thus blocking caffeine action. Tertiary amine
local anesthetics, in their uncharged form, act in a manner very
similar to caffeine; that is, one can produce a contracture with
these agents. Therefore, one has a balance between two sites of
action with regard to tertiary amine local anesthetics. In the surface membrane, these agents can decrease excitability and reduce
the action potential, thereby producing relaxation by uncoupling or
preventing the exciting event from occurring. But in the sarcoplasmic reticulum (where, in their charged form, agents with the
carbonyl group would tend to antagonize the action of caffeine)
tertiary amines, in their uncharged form, seem to act in a manner
similar to caffeine.

In lidocaine (Xylocaine), an anesthetic which has two methyl
groups in the ortho positions and has an association constant

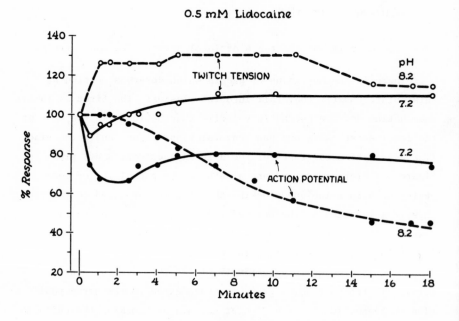

FIG. 3.   Effect of sub-blocking dose of lidocaine on action
potential and twitch tension.

for H+ of 7.95 (pKa): at physiological pH, we have a good balance
between both the charged and uncharged forms.

Figure 3 illustrates the way in which a sub-blocking dose of
lidocaine affects action potential and twitch tension as a function
of pH. With a pH of 7.2, the action potential is initially very
markedly decreased and then slowly returns to a level which is maintained at about 80% of the initial response. This type of response
is correlated more with the uptake and redistribution of the lidocaine in the muscle fiber at this pH. However, if one looks at
twitch tension, one sees associated with the initial rapid drop
first a decrease, then a slow return and maintenance of the twitch
at about its 100% level, even though the action potential has been
decreased by 20%. If we raise the pH to produce more of the uncharged form of lidocaine, we notice a depression of the action
potential and yet a marked potentiation of the twitch—up to the
point where close to 60% or 40% of the potential spike is depressed.
Here we begin to have a block of the twitch as a function of
the decrease in the action potential; that is, there can be a decrease of the monophastic action potential amplitude, down to
around 30% of its maximum, before it affects the coupling event.
This shows that the action of lidocaine, whether on the sarcolemmal
membrane with regard to action potential or on the sarcoplasmic
reticulum with regard to the calcium stores, is a function of the
nature of its charge.

I'd like to turn to some work that Dr. George Strobel (5,6)
has recently done which is related to the interaction between
Halothane, forane, and caffeine. The basis of these studies is
related to the condition known as malignant hyperthermia, in which
it is believed thereis a pharmacogenetic defect of the sarcoplasmic
reticulum. In this condition, when halothane is used as an anesthetic, there is a decrease in the ability of the sarcoplasmic
reticulum to retain calcium. It can take up calcium, we believe,
but it cannot retain it. Therefore it's equivalent to having a
constant turnover of calcium. ATP restores it to the longitudinal

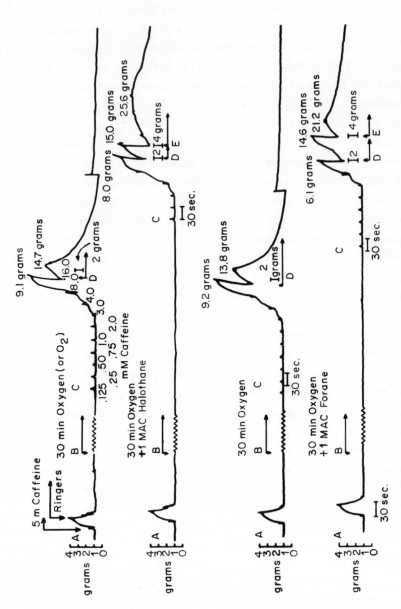

FIG. 4. Experimental simulation of malignant hyperthemic lesion in sartorius muscle.

reticulum, but it cannot be retained in the terminal cisterni. This
results in a marked rigidity (increase in contracture), a marked
rise in temperature, and a dramatic breakdown of muscle mass and
muscle tissue. It's a very explosive event, and it's triggered by
the volatile anesthetic. Experimentally, we can take the sartorius
muscle and produce a contracture similar in type to the lesion
caused by the administration of halothane (Fig. 3). The control
response for 5 mM caffeine is on the left (Fig. 4); the contracture
is reversible and the caffeine contractures are within 5% of each
other on paired muscles. After 30 minutes of recovery in oxygen,
a cumulative-dose-response curve to caffeine is obtained. Each
curve represents a timed cumulative-dose-response curve in which
every 30 seconds the caffeine concentration is increased. From 0.125
mM to 3 mM caffeine no tension is observed. One minimum alveolar
concentration (MAC) of halothane, which is equivalent to what would

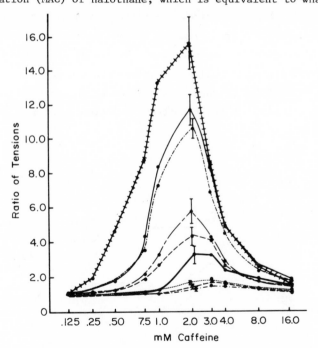

FIG. 5.   Effectiveness of volatile anesthetics in potentiating
caffeine contracture.

be used to produce anesthesia in man, causes a marked dramatic
increase in tension.

In Figure 5 Dr. Strobel has plotted a series of volatile
anesthetics, using always their MAC required for anesthesia. What
Figure 5 illustrates is that chloroform is most effective in potentiating a caffeine contracture. In the presence of the volatile
anesthetic and various caffeine concentrations, the ratio of tension development is plotted. We see that chloroform is very
effective. Halothane is next, followed by penthrane, then ethrane.
Least effective were forane and ether. The safest volatile anesthetics, with regard to this type of lesion produced in a muscle
by caffeine, are ether, forane and nitrous oxide. We have seen
that there are dramatic differences among volatile anesthetics
regarding contracture produced in skeletal muscle. One agent that
has been used successfully to overcome the effects of malignant
hyperthermia is procainamide. In relatively high concentrations
it has reversed the condition and ensured patient survival (6).
One would caution very much against the use of lidocaine under these
conditions. Since lidocaine in skeletal muscle acts in a manner
similar to caffeine, lidocaine would not be the best choice of
local anesthetic with which to treat a patient with malignant
hyperthermia.

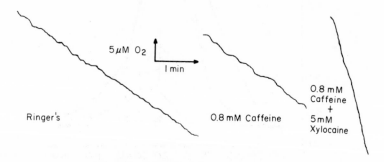

FIG. 6. Interactive effect of Xylocaine (lidocaine) and
caffeine on rate of oxygen uptake.

Figure 6 illustrates a second aspect of calcium; that is, involvement in what we call excitation-respiration coupling. Here
again we see an interaction between the local anesthetic, lidocaine
(Xylocaine) and caffeine; but it is no longer producing tension.
What we are measuring is an increase in the rate of oxygen consumption. This is the work that Novotny and I did back in 1966 (7).
What we see is that 0.8 mM caffeine by itself has no effect on the
rate of oxygen uptake. However, if lidocaine is added to the 0.8
mM caffeine, there is a marked dramatic increase in oxygen intake.
This action is very suggestive of malignant hyperthermia. In 70%
of the cases the increased muscle metabolism is associated with
rigidity; in the remaining cases increased metabolism is not associated with rigidity, even though one gets the dramatic rise in
body temperature. This suggests that the level of calcium within
the muscle fiber will determine whether tension develops or

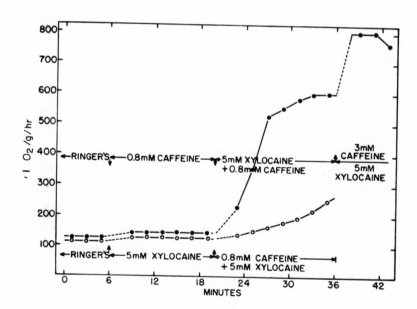

FIG. 7. Effect of caffeine-Xylocaine sequence of administration on rate of oxygen uptake.

whether an increase in the metabolic rate develops due to the stimulation of the system that leads to an increase in oxygen uptake.

Caffeine contracture is not produced at 0.8 mM caffeine, but the increase of respiration (oxygen uptake) depends upon the sequence with which one gives the caffeine (Fig. 7). In the upper black dots we go into Ringer solution and prime the muscle with 0.8 mM caffeine. If lidocaine is added to the caffeine there is a dramatic increase in oxygen uptake. Increasing the caffeine further increases oxygen uptake. If the lidocaine is administered first, and then the caffeine, there takes place, instead of a dramatic sharp rise, a slow rate of increase. Therefore, there is an effect at this low level of caffeine even though it did not produce any effect on oxygen uptake. However, it did lead to a modification of response once the lidocaine was added. The response in the presence of caffeine is not lost when external calcium is removed. Therefore, the calcium that is required for this system to operate comes from the sarcoplasmic reticulum and is thus supplied from inside. Since there is no tension developed under these conditions, the level of calcium required to stimulate this system must be on the order of 10^{-7} M (we believe it to be between 10^{-9} and 10^{-7}).

If we look at the other method for coupling excitation to respiration, that is, potassium depolarization, we observe that lidocaine at 5 mM produces a marked increase in the oxygen consumption at 12.5 mM. If we go to 18 mM KCl, there is a further increase but not as marked. We seem to approach a saturation level. Now, these levels of potassium depolarization are all below the threshold for contraction. What one sees under these conditions is a sustained increase in calcium influx, and it is this system that is markedly affected by the removal of external calcium. Uncoupling can take place, and if nickel or another divalent ion (with the exception of magnesium) is present it can replace the calcium involved in this coupling system.

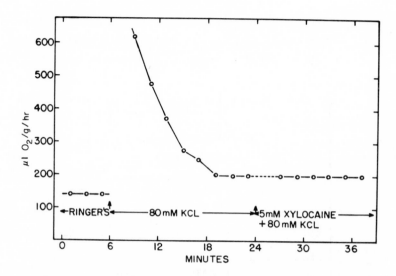

FIG. 8.   Xylocaine, potassium depolarization, and oxygen consumption.

The action of lidocaine is associated with an event that takes place during the initial triggering step, as indicated by the fact that when 80 mM KCl is added there is a phasic contracture which lasts only about 3 minutes. Oxygen uptake shows a marked increase and then declines to a steady level over a 15-minute period. This level is above baseline and is associated with the recovery heat (Fig. 8). I'd like to point out that our concern here is the coupling step with regard to depolarization below the level at which tension is developed in the muscle.

The next work is that of Joan Dawson, and is extracted from the thesis for which she received her Ph.D. (8). The background for the work is as follows. In our laboratory we've been working with the glycerol-treated preparation in terms of what effect glycerol treatment would have on calcium flux. What we observed in the course of our experiments is that in glycerol treatment (a procedure whereby a muscle was put into a hypertonic glycerol, 400 mM, and allowed to recover in normal Ringer solution for 60 minutes) glycerol distributed itself across the membrane, increasing

the osmolarity inside the muscle fiber such that when it was returned to a normal Ringer solution, it was markedly hypertonic to
the sarcoplasm. Hence water was taken up, the muscle fiber swelled,

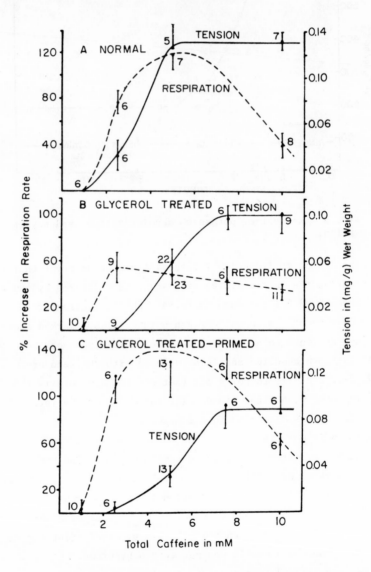

FIG. 9. Effect of caffeine on respiration-contraction of
glycerol-treated muscle.

and during the course of this swelling a disruption of about 80 to
90% of the transverse tubular elements occurred. The major effect
was an uncoupling between electrical stimulation—even though there
was an action potential, it could no longer stimulate the contraction. If one depolarizes with potassium in a muscle treated
in this manner, there is no contraction. If one depolarizes and
measures oxygen uptake, which Van der Kloot did, one observes no
coupling between potassium depolarization and respiration (9).
Therefore both systems are uncoupled in glycerol-treated muscle
fibers.

We noticed that the magnesium content fell from a value of
about 9 $\mu M/g$ as a control to about 4.5 $\mu M/g$ in the glycerol-treated
muscle. This indicated a marked reduction in the magnesium content
of the muscle fiber. We initially thought that perhaps the reason
potassium depolarization and respiration could be uncoupled was
due to the low magnesium content. Joan Dawson then undertook the
study of what factors were involved in the uncoupling of the excitation-respiration response in glycerol-treated muscle, and whether
magnesium or a caffeine release of calcium could overcome the defect. In the top curve of Figure 9 we see the control response.
That is, the dotted line indicates the rise in respiration in the
control as a function of caffeine concentration. This was 2 mM
up to 10 mM. There was a marked increase in oxygen uptake even
though the amount of tension developed was small. At peak contracture tension there was a decrease in oxygen uptake. We believe
that this decrease is an area for subsequent research. We're only
concerned at this point with the events which occur in the region
below tension development.

The glycerol-treated muscle in which we uncoupled excitation
and contraction and excitation and respiration could produce a
respiratory response to caffeine, but compared to the control it
was markedly reduced, whereas the tension was very close to what
it was in untreated muscles, although there was a slight shift to
higher caffeine concentrations. In an experiment in which the

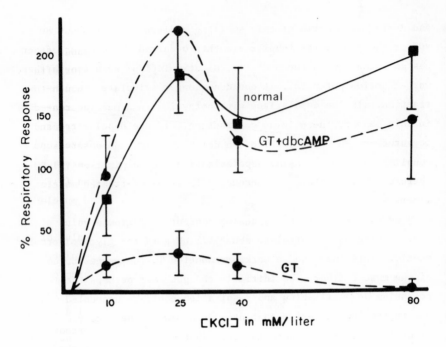

FIG. 10. Effect of dbcAMP on potassium stimulation of
GT muscle.

glycerol-treated muscle is primed by adding 1 mM caffeine (theophylline can be used as well), as the caffeine concentration is
increased there is an increase in the oxygen consumption. Therefore, it appears that the glycerol-treated muscle, when it is
primed with an inhibitor of phosphodiesterase, is liable to dramatically increased excitation-respiration. Caffeine stimulation
of respiration is not affected by the removal of external calcium.
However, calcium is required for potassium stimulation of respiration. As external potassium concentration is increased there is a
slight rise in oxygen uptake not significantly different from the
baseline (Fig. 10). This slight rise, however, I feel is a real
one, because in a glycerol-treated muscle not all of the transverse
tubular elements are disrupted; there is a small fraction which is

maintained intact and which may account for the slight rise in
baseline. If one adds to the treated muscle dibutyryl cyclic AMP
or cyclic AMP, the potassium stimulation of respiration is restored.
The addition of procaine will block excitation-respiration, while
the removal of external calcium will block potassium-stimulated
respiration. In a glycerol-treated muscle without dibutyryl cyclic
AMP there is an increase in calcium influx, but no increase in
respiration associated with potassium depolarization.

Both calcium and cyclic AMP appear to be involved in the respiratory response and the coupling step. Prostaglandin E_1 causes a
marked increase in oxygen uptake when applied before caffeine.
Polyphoretin phosphate dramatically reduces the respiratory response
of normal muscle to potassium, but enhances the potassium contracture. Clearly, excitation-respiration and excitation-contracture
coupling are parallel, but serial, events; and one can demonstrate
that both of these events can be uncoupled.

In summary, we have shown that calcium is involved in two
coupling processes in muscle. Calcium and cyclic AMP appear to be
involved in the excitation and respiration of glycerol-treated
muscles. The calcium that acts at this site is within the region
of 10^{-9} to 10^{-7} M. We believe calcium acts at an internal site,
since calcium released from sarcoplasmic reticulum can stimulate
the response. One can replace calcium with nickel or other divalent ions (except magnesium) for this coupling process. For the
coupling process involved in contraction only barium and strontium
can replace the calcium, and calcium is required at between 10^{-7}
and 10^{-6} M.

Local anesthetics, depending on whether they are charged or
uncharged, will modify the system. Lidocaine will enhance contraction, and unlike its effect on brain tissue, where it blocks a
potassium respiration response (as does procaine), it enhances the
respiratory response of muscle to external potassium.

REFERENCES

1. L. L. Costantin, J. Gen. Physiol., 55: 703 (1970).

2. E. X. Albuquerque, J. E. Warnick, and F. M. Sansone, J. Pharmacol. Exp. Ther., 176: 511 (1971).

3. J. N. Howell and D. J. Jenden, Fed. Proc. Fed. Amer. Soc. Exp. Biol., 26: 553 (1967).

4. G. Strobel, unpublished work, 1973.

5. G. Strobel and C. P. Bianchi, Anesthesiology, 35: 465 (1971).

6. B. A. Britt, in "Symposium on Metabolic Effects of Anesthesia," Royal College of Surgeons, London, Sept., 1970.

7. I. Novotny and C. P. Bianchi, J. Pharmacol. and Exp. Ther., 155: 456 (1967).

8. M. J. Dawson and C. P. Bianchi, Eur. J. Pharmacol., 30: 288 (1975).

9. W. Van der Kloot, J. Physiol. (London), 204: 551 (1969).

Chapter 14

CALCIUM AND THE SARCOPLASMIC RETICULUM

Anthony H. Caswell

Department of Pharmacology
University of Miami School of Medicine
Miami, Florida

Very few drugs exert their therapeutic action directly on the sarcoplasmic reticulum. On the other hand, very many drugs exert their action in determining internal Ca^{2+} availability. However, we do not know how Ca^{2+} is released from these stores and made available to the contractile apparatus. Because we do not know this, it is very difficult to evaluate the actions of many of the drugs which we see used therapeutically.

What I want to do is simply to present an idea. It is a simple idea, but it's a general one about the nature of excitation-contraction coupling. First I want to describe very briefly some of the experiments I've been doing which gave rise to this postulate. And then I'll describe the postulate itself.

I've been working on isolated sarcoplasmic reticulum (SR) from rabbit skeletal muscle, employing fluorescent chelate probes as a means of observing Ca^{2+} movements into and out of the SR. With the probe technique we introduce the reagent, chlorotetracycline, which fluoresces with great intensity when it binds with Ca^{2+} on a membrane surface. The initial external Ca^{2+} concentration is very low, and very little Ca^{2+} is bound to the membrane surface. But when it is accumulated within the SR, the concentration of Ca^{2+} within the vesicle rises to a high level, and a substantial portion

of this is bound to the membrane surface. Chlorotetracycline is
able to penetrate within a membrane and will then bind to the Ca^{2+}
on the membrane surface. One can observe the events, then, of Ca^{2+}
accumulation by isolated SR as an increase in the fluorescence of
chlorotetracycline.

The nature of the data which one obtains is illustrated in
Figure 1. SR is present in the system, as is chlorotetracycline.
If the uptake of Ca^{2+} is initiated by the addition of ATP, one sees
an initial decrease in fluorescence which is due to chelation of
Mg^{2+} present in the medium to ATP. Following this, a rise in the
fluorescence is observed associated with the uptake of Ca^{2+}. That

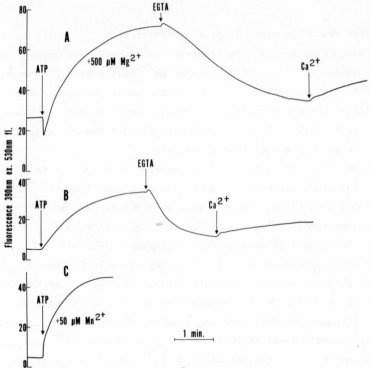

FIG. 1. Visualization of Ca^{2+} accumulation by SR using chlorotetracycline as a fluorescent chelate probe. Media consisted of
50 mM histidine, 350 mM sucrose, 10 µM chlorotetracycline, SR 0.30
mg protein/ml. pH was 6.8 and temperature 22°. Additions to the
media were: ATP, 500 µM; Tris EGTA, 500 µM; $CaCl_2$, 100 µM.

this is indeed a measure of Ca^{2+} accumulation is demonstrated by the subsequent addition of EGTA, which chelates external Ca^{2+}. This creates an increased Ca^{2+} gradient and causes the Ca^{2+} release which is associated in Figure 1 with a diminution in the fluorescence of chlorotetracycline. The effect can be subsequently reversed by further addition of Ca^{2+}. The other traces simply show what happens if Mg^{2+} is omitted, in which case there occurs a smaller increase in the fluorescence associated with a less efficient accumulation of Ca^{2+}. This illustrates that Mg^{2+} is a required cofactor for the ATP stimulated Ca^{2+} uptake. It is possible to replace Mg^{2+} with Mn^{2+} and retain high Ca^{2+} accumulation. This is shown in Figure 1C.

Recently I've been trying to repeat some of the work of Makinose and Hasselbach (1), who have shown that it is possible to reverse the Ca^{2+} pump using the techniques described above. This is shown in Figure 2. A technique for observing the release of Ca^{2+} associated with ATP synthesis is to add EGTA after Ca^{2+} has been allowed to accumulate. The EGTA binds to external Ca^{2+}, which creates an electrochemical gradient of Ca^{2+} higher than the phosphate potential of ATP. This should cause release of Ca^{2+}. For reversal of the Ca^{2+} pump, ADP and Pi are required as substrates and ATP is synthesized during Ca^{2+} release. In Figure 2 the release of Ca^{2+} is observed showing the substrate specificity of the reversal of the pump. In this figure, in the presence of isolated SR, ATP causes Ca^{2+} accumulation. The addition of ADP causes a certain Ca^{2+} release which is presumably associated with the fact that the chemical potential of ATP is reduced by addition of ADP. The subsequent addition of EGTA causes a rapid Ca^{2+} release. The substrate specificity is shown in Figures 2B, C, and D. If ADP is omitted, a rapid release of Ca^{2+} still occurs, but this is not surprising, since ADP is being formed from the breakdown of ATP during Ca^{2+} accumulation. So in order to eliminate ADP, the reaction has been coupled to creatinine phosphokinase and creatinine phosphate in such a way that any ADP formed during Ca^{2+} accumulation would be immediately converted back to ATP (Fig. 2C). In this way it is possible to eliminate ADP from the system. Under these conditions,

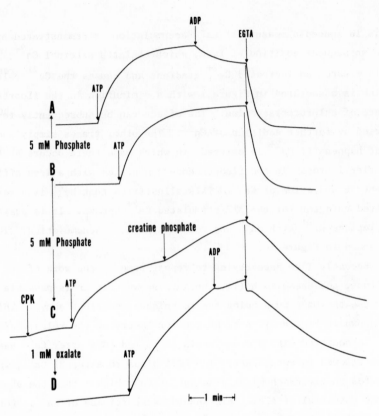

FIG. 2. Release of Ca^{2+} from SR facilitated by ADP and Pi.
Media contained: 5 mM histidine, 200 mM sucrose, 50 mM KCl, 1 mM
$MgCl_2$, 100 µM $CaCl_2$, 10 µM chlorotetracycline. pH was 6.8 and
temperature 22°. Additions to the media were: ATP, 200 µM; ADP,
1 mM; EGTA, 1 mM; creatinine phosphate, 1 mM.

if EGTA is added subsequently, then the release of Ca^{2+} is very
much slower, indicating a requirement for ADP in the release process. Similarly, if Pi is replaced with oxalate or Cl' the addition of EGTA again causes a slow release of Ca^{2+} (Fig. 2D). The
rapidity of the reversal of the Ca^{2+} pump is indeed striking.
Thus, the pump is extremely reversible and release occurs within a
few seconds. This is the same time period as that for Ca^{2+} accumulation in isolated SR. It occurred to me then that it was possible
that the process of excitation-contraction coupling could cause
Ca^{2+} release through the same enzyme system as that for Ca^{2+} uptake.
The question then arose, how could this process be triggered?

A number of hypotheses have been made concerning the nature of excitation-contraction coupling. It has been proposed that specific transmitters are released by the T tubules. Ford and Podolsky (2) have shown that a pulse of Ca^{2+} ions given to skinned muscle fibers may induce release of Ca^{2+} from SR. Nakamaru and Schwartz (3) have proposed that a pulse of H^+ ions initiates Ca^{2+} release. On the other hand, experiments have been conducted to demonstrate that Ca^{2+} release by SR is initiated by a depolarization of the SR membrane (2,4,5). The means of effecting depolarization has been to increase the concentrations of Cl' in the cytoplasm. Such experiments might be subjected to artifactual considerations, since Carvalho and Leo (6) have demonstrated that when SR is incubated in high KCl, the KCl enters the SR matrix and competes for binding sites with Ca^{2+}, thus causing Ca^{2+} release. Thus it may be considered that experimental information is not currently adequate to distinguish or identify the true mechanism of Ca^{2+} release by SR.

If one actually considers what happens inside the intact muscle, one thing which is rather noteworthy is the fact that there are two subcellular organelles within the muscle fibers, both of which have identical substrate requirements. These are the myofibrils and the SR. Both require Ca^{2+} and ATP for activity. In the case of the SR, ATP breakdown occurs only when Ca^{2+} is present in the cytoplasm. This gives rise, then, to Ca^{2+} accumulation by the SR and the loss of Ca^{2+} from the cytoplasm. In the case of the myofibrils the actomyosin ATPase, again, is activated in the presence of Ca^{2+}. And thus we have a situation in which two organelles are both competing for the same substrates. When such a situation exists, there is the possibility of a biological switch. A biological switch, then, is associated with two stable or metastable states. Once a trigger has been applied which has driven the system from one stable state, it will automatically move through an unstable state to a second stable state. The question is: How could this happen in muscle? It is possible according to the data of Ford and Podolsky (2) that cytoplasmic Ca^{2+} is the source of the trigger for contraction.

The initial relaxed state is such that the cytoplasmic Ca^{2+} is low, the myofibrillar ATPase is low, the SR ATPase is low, and Ca^{2+} within the SR is high. When the muscle is excited, the excitation wave may pass down the T tubules and cause Ca^{2+} movement from the extracellular space or from internal stores into the cytoplasm. If this Ca^{2+} binds to the myofibrils, it will initiate an increased ATPase. As soon as ATP is broken down the equilibrium between the electrochemical potential of the Ca^{2+} gradient across the SR on

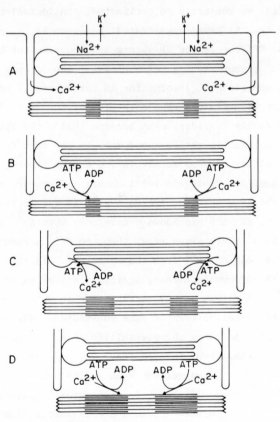

FIG. 3.   Diagrammatic concept of biological switch in muscle contraction.

the one hand and the phosphate potential of ATP on the other will
be destroyed. As ATP is hydrolyzed, the phosphate potential will
drop. There will be a tendency then for Ca^{2+} to be released from
the SR. As soon as Ca^{2+} is released from the SR it will bind to
troponin and activate the myofibrillar ATPase. This in turn will
cause the phosphate potential of ATP to drop further. As the phosphate potential declines still further, more Ca^{2+} will be released
from the SR in an attempt to readjust the equilibrium. This is the
concept of the biological switch. This is illustrated diagrammatically in Figure 3.

What stops this process? A new quasistable state will be
reached when the phosphate potential of ATP is no longer below that
of the equilibrium potential of the Ca^{2+} gradient across the SR.
The ATP level will become balanced on the one hand by the hydro-
lytic reaction of the myofibrillar ATPase and on the other by the
synthetic reactions of the creatine phosphokinase and the mito-
chondrial energy conservation process. The final steady state will
not necessarily involve total release of Ca^{2+} from the SR.

How does the muscle relax? It is not clear at this stage how
the trigger process for the relaxation can occur. However, once
relaxation is started, it has to continue until the muscle reverts
back to the relaxed state. The initiation of the reverse process
occurs if by any mechanism the phosphate potential of ATP transi-
torily rises above the equilibrium potential of Ca^{2+} across the
SR, because as soon as that occurs there has to be an uptake of
Ca^{2+} into the SR. However, following the uptake of Ca^{2+} into the
SR, the myofibrillar ATPase will be reduced. This is caused by a
diminution in the cytoplasmic Ca^{2+} concentration. Therefore the
balance between the creatine phosphokinase and the myofibrillar
ATPase would be altered in favor of ATP synthesis. Hence the
phosphate potential of ATP will rise still further. And the rise
in the phosphate potential will be associated with further uptake
of Ca^{2+} into the SR. Then a cascade process will occur in reverse

RELAXATION

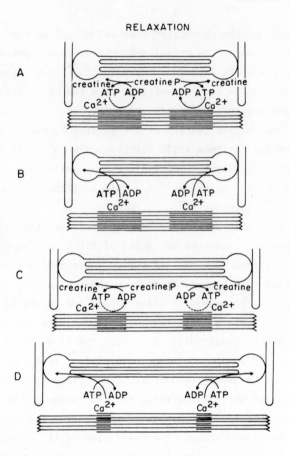

FIG. 4.   Diagrammatic concept of muscle relaxation.

until complete relaxation has occurred.   Figure 4 shows this
concept diagrammatically.

This proposed mechanism of excitation-contraction coupling
incorporates facets of muscle action which are already understood
and described.   No further assumptions concerning the physiology or
biochemistry of muscle components are made.   It also opens the
possibility for experiments to be devised to test the hypothesis.
These are currently under consideration.   I propose this hypothesis
in the spirit of enquiry rather than of commitment.

REFERENCES

1. M. Makinese and W. Hasselbach, Fed. Eur. Biochem. Soc. Lett.,
    12: 271 (1971).

2. L. E. Ford and R. J. Podolsky, J. Physiol. (London), 223: 1,
    (1972).

3. Y. Nakamaru and A. Schwartz, J. Gen. Physiol., 59: 22 (1972).

4. M. Endo and J. R. Blinks, Nature New Biol., 246: 220 (1973).

5. M. Casai and H. Miyamoto, Fed. Eur. Biochem. Soc. Lett.,
    34: 299 (1973).

6. A. P. Carvalho and B. Leo, J. Gen. Physiol., 50: 1327 (1967).

Chapter 15

CALCIUM AND SMOOTH MUSCLE

Andrew P. Somlyo

Department of Physiology and Pathology
Presbyterian-University of Pennsylvania Medical Center
Philadelphia, Pennsylvania

Since the title of this paper indicates a relatively restricted subject, it might not be altogether superfluous to mention that, in a broader context, smooth muscle plays a rather major role in clinical pharmacology. To illustrate this point, I shall merely note that oxytocic and antihypertensive agents, as well as drugs used to treat acute asthmatic attacks, really act by contracting or relaxing smooth muscle (1). And, as I shall further attempt to show, they do so by modifying cellular calcium levels (2). The specificity of the response of smooth muscle to different drugs will be keyed by tissue specific factors—such as receptors, second messengers and ionic equilibrium potentials—as well as the specific nature of the drug. For example, the cholinergic drugs will tend to contract intestinal smooth muscle, whereas they will relax the peripheral vascular bed and produce vasodilation.

Specificity of contractile versus relaxant effects, therefore, is not always keyed to a given drug. In other words, it's very seldom possible to say that one drug is a smooth-muscle excitatory agent and another one an inhibitory agent. With the exception of β-adrenergic action, which generally tends to be relaxant (1,3),

This chapter was transcribed from a tape recording of the Second Annual Clinical Pharmacology Symposium held in Key Biscayne, Florida, March 7-10, 1973.

for most active smooth-muscle agents you will find an example where
one smooth muscle will be excited and the other one inhibited by
the same drug. Similarly, even different portions of the same
blood vessel may react differentially to the same drug. For example, in some species the sensitivity of the aorta to vasopressin
increases caudally, from a total absence of vasopressin sensitivity
in the thoracic aorta to rather considerable sensitivity near the
bifurcation.

The definition of smooth muscle is an old, light microscopic
one, and I shall begin by showing what smooth muscle is not. On
the first slide you see a phase-interference light micrograph of a
single striated-muscle fiber, with the sarcomeres (striations) delineated by Z lines. The micropipette loaded with calcium was
applied to the slightly injured surface membrane of the fiber,
causing a local contracture, illustrated by the narrowing of the
sarcomere pattern. This, as well as most of the difficult experiments that I shall discuss today, were done by Avril Somlyo. The
next slide is a phase-interference micrograph of a single smooth-
muscle fiber. This is the single fiber preparation (4,5) from toad
stomach that is rather easy to disperse. There is no evidence of
the striations that you see in the striated muscle, hence the name
smooth muscle.

Nevertheless, when you stimulate these smooth-muscle fibers, as
you see on the next slide, the fibers can shorten and shorten remarkably, as of course is well known about the whole muscle. As a
matter of fact, the total shortening of the smooth-muscle fibers,
in this case stimulated by acetylcholine, is greater than 50% of
the initial muscle length (5). This, in fact, is in excess of
what one could expect on the basis of a conventional sarcomere
arrangement such as you see in striated muscles.

What I would like to consider is the question of how the contraction is initiated in smooth muscle in general; how calcium plays
a role in the initiation and maintenance of this contraction; and
finally, what the contractile mechanism is that is activated by
calcium. As has been earlier pointed out by Paul Bianchi, striated-
muscle contraction (twitch) is initiated by an action potential.

This releases calcium from the terminal cisternae of the sarcoplasmic reticulum. The initiation of contraction in smooth muscle
may be either by an action potential, such as you see on this slide,
or by some other process, which I shall discuss later (6,7). In
this slide, the upper trace is the electrical and the lower trace
the mechanical record of the activity of the rabbit portal vein.
This particular smooth muscle, like several visceral smooth muscles
(e.g., taenia coli and estrogen-treated uterus), generates spontaneous action potentials that trigger twitch contractions. In
response to an excitatory agent, in this case norepinephrine, there
is an increase in the frequency of the action potentials and in
tension: this record is by definition a tetanus, high-frequency
spike discharge with fused mechanical activity.

It was argued some years ago that perhaps the charge carried by
the action potential is calcium, and that this calcium activates
the twitch itself. More recently, this hypothesis has been proven
incorrect, because the charge carried by the action potential, even
if it were a pure calcium current, could not be sufficient to activate the contractile process. Furthermore, the evidence, limited
thus far to uterine muscle, suggests that not the whole charge but
only a fraction of it is perhaps carried by calcium, the remainder
being carried by sodium. Nevertheless, we are left with the question of how these action potentials trigger the twitch contractions
in this type of smooth muscle.

Increasing the concentration of the stimulatory agents produces
further depolarization, in which the action potentials are wiped
out and the membrane is electrically quiet. The tension record
shown here, in response to a high concentration of norepinephrine,
is a contracture (without associated action potentials) such as
occurs also in some slow tonic striated muscles (for example, the
iliofibularis bundle of the frog and the latissimus dorsi of the
pigeon).

The response of intestinal smooth muscle to acetylcholine is
similar, and the fundamental process of electromechanical coupling

probably is the same. Stimulating drugs at low concentrations produce some depolarization and increased frequency of action-potential
discharge; at higher concentrations the drugs produce further depolarization and, usually, tension.

Action potentials, however, are not the only type of electrical
response of smooth muscle to drugs. Other types of smooth muscles,
illustrated on this slide, respond to excitation by a graded depolarization without action potentials (6,7). This example is of
smooth muscle in the main pulmonary artery of the rabbit. The
upper trace is the electrical and the lower trace the mechanical
record. In response to a low concentration of norepinephrine the
membrane depolarizes, but there is not the burst of action potentials shown earlier by the portal vein. An increase in the concentration of the excitatory agent leads to greater depolarization.
This type of muscle is found in large arteries. The canine trach-
ealis smooth muscle also responds with graded depolarization, a
process rather similar to the end-plate potential. Graded depolarization and action potentials are two types of electromechanical
coupling, but they are not the only mechanisms of drug-induced
excitation of smooth muscle.

Even when the membrane potential of smooth muscles is abolished,
by placing them in a high potassium solution, stimulating agents
can still elicit contractions (6,8). It is also possible to produce relaxation of such depolarized muscles with agents such as
isoproterenol. Illustrated here are the contractile responses of
aortic strips to three different stimulating agents: angiotensin,
vasopressin and epinephrine (6). The preparations have been depolarized with a high potassium solution prior to the beginning of
the experiment to eliminate all the membrane-potential-mediated
responses. Nevertheless, these drugs can still produce contractions.
There is an aspect of this experiment that is unique to smooth muscle and not found in striated muscles: the maximal contractions
produced on the same smooth-muscle strip by the different stimulating agents are unequal. For example, no matter how much

angiotensin we add beyond a certain concentration, this particular smooth muscle will contract only partially; this response is much less than the maximal response to epinephrine. These experiments also illustrate an important aspect of the clinical pharmacology of smooth muscle; that is, they respond and are regulated by a variety of neurotransmitters, hormones, physiological and pathological agents. In contrast, mammalian striated muscles are normally excited by a single neurotransmitter, acetylcholine.

The question then arises, What does all this have to do with calcium? Implied in this discussion will be the assumption that calcium initiates the contraction as a second messenger, to use the current vernacular, whether it is triggered by an action potential, by graded depolarization, or by pharmacomechanical coupling, a process not controlled by a change in membrane potential. The evidence for the role of calcium stems from several types of experiments, and primarily those that show that glycerinated smooth muscles are contracted and smooth-muscle actomyosin ATPase is activated by calcium (2). This glycerination is not the type of experiment that Paul Bianchi spoke about. Rather, the muscle is placed in a 50% glycerol solution for up to several months so that the membrane, nearly completely destroyed, becomes very leaky. Therefore, very low concentrations of externally applied agents that would not permeate the normal membrane can interact with the regulatory proteins. In such experiments, as buffered calcium is added to glycerinated smooth muscle, ATPase activity and tension is activated between $10^{-7}M - 10^{-5}M$ calcium. In general, we may then assume that, no matter how the electrical or nonelectrical (pharmacomechanical) mechanism is involved in the activation of smooth-muscle contraction, the final common activator step is the rise in intracellular free-calcium concentration.

One may increase the intracellular free-calcium concentration even in nonglycerinated muscle, if the muscle is depolarized with a high potassium solution, but the concentrations required are considerably higher than for the glycerinated muscle. Apparently, the

permeability of the nonglycerinated membrane to calcium is relatively low even in the depolarized state. Nevertheless, such experiments suggest that extracellular calcium may be one source for
contractile activation of smooth muscle. This question will be
dealt with by Casey van Breeman in terms of calcium fluxes, and I
shall only note here that agents that decrease transmembrane calcium flux, such as the local anesthetics, can inhibit this kind of
contraction. The experiment shown here illustrates the dose-
dependent and reversible relaxation of the potassium-calcium contracture by procaine (7). The relaxation of the muscle, as well as
its contraction upon removal of procaine from the depolarized
muscle contracted by calcium, are a little more rapid in the rabbit
mesenteric vein than in the aorta.

This type of experiment certainly indicates one possible source
of calcium that can activate smooth muscle. Stimulation of transmembrane calcium movements by excitatory drugs can also be tested
by another type of experiment, by measuring the electrical responses
(depolarization) to stimulatory agents while the muscles are bathed
in a solution in which the primary extracellular cation is calcium
(a sodium-free solution). Making certain assumptions about anion
fluxes, one assumes under these conditions that depolarization is at
least a semiquantitative measure of the inward calcium movement
caused by the excitatory agent.

Experiments on rabbit main-pulmonary-artery smooth muscle in
such (sodium-free) solutions show that supramaximal concentrations
of serotonin depolarize the muscles, suggesting that there is some
increase in calcium permeability (9). Addition of norepinephrine
produces further depolarization, suggesting that the effect of
norepinephrine on calcium permeability is greater than that of
serotonin. The maximal contraction produced by serotonin is also
less than that elicited by norepinephrine. These experiments suggest that the changes in membrane permeability are proportional to
the magnitude of the maximal contractions stimulated by different
drugs. I will hasten to add, however, that the activation of

muscle cannot be explained solely by transmembrane calcium
fluxes.

The next question was how to localize intracellular calcium
stores, if they are present in smooth muscle. In striated muscle,
intracellular calcium is stored primarily in the sarcoplasmic reticulum. We therefore used electron microscopic techniques to
examine the ultrastructure of smooth muscle (10,11). In sections
of longitudinal smooth muscle of rabbit portal vein, there are
some tubular elements of sarcoplasmic reticulum. However, the
amount of sarcoplasmic reticulum in this muscle is rather scanty.
It is perhaps not surprising that earlier electron microscopists,
who used different fixatives that tended to damage the sarcoplasmic reticulum, felt that there was no, or only a very rudimentary,
sarcoplasmic reticulum in smooth muscle. However, in physiologi-
cally different types of smooth muscle, such as the main pulmonary
artery, the sarcoplasmic reticulum is much more prominent. In such
muscles ribosomes are also more often found on the tubules, indicating that part of the sacroplasmic reticulum is a rough endoplas-
mic reticulum. This is possible evidence of protein synthesis.
There is now good evidence from both tissue-culture studies and experiments on intact aorta, that the smooth muscle of the large arteries also synthesizes the extracellular proteins, collagen and
elastin (12). It is probable that the presence of large amounts of
sarcoplasmic reticulum is indicative of the type of smooth muscle
that is engaged in protein synthesis. Proliferation of the sarcoplasmic reticulum is one of the most common nonspecific signs of
injury to smooth muscle and, therefore, one speculates whether injury may also incidentally increase the cellular calcium stores of
smooth muscles (10,13).

The rabbit aorta, the favorite tool of smooth-muscle pharmacologists, also contains relatively large amounts of sarcoplasmic
reticulum (11). Stacked elements of these tubular structures are
often found in the smooth muscle of aortic and main pulmonary artery.

In longitudinal sections there is often a rather characteristic appearance of sarcoplasmic reticulum in all types of smooth muscle studied, including portal vein and turtle oviduct (10,11). It consists of tubules of the sarcoplasmic reticulum fenestrated around the surface (plasmalemmal) vesicles.

If the tubular elements are sarcoplasmic reticulum, then they should not directly communicate with the extracellular space either in or outside the plane of a given section. Indeed, it has been shown by using extracellular tracers (ferritin, colloidal lanthanum, horseradish peroxidase) (10,11) that these tubules do not communicate with the extracellular space, but are a true sarcoplasmic reticulum. The extracellular markers enter the surface vesicles, indicating that they communicate with the extracellular space, as do, for example, the T tubules of striated muscle. Ferritin particles do not enter the fenestrated tubules encircling the vesicles nor the other tubules that, by these criteria at least, constitute a true closed tubular system of sarcoplasmic reticulum.

We are next faced with the question of how an action potential, traveling along the surface membrane, triggers the release of calcium presumably stored in the sarcoplasmic reticulum. In skeletal muscle there are contacts between the terminal cisternae of the sarcoplasmic reticulum and the invaginated surface membrane of the T tubules. In smooth muscle and in some cardiac muscles, the sites of contact are between elements of the surface membrane not invaginated and the adjacent junctional sarcoplasmic reticulum. High magnification views show periodic (every 200 to 250 $\overset{\circ}{A}$) densities traversing the 100 to 120 $\overset{\circ}{A}$ space between the sarcoplasmic reticulum and the surface membrane of smooth muscles. The entire complex resembles the couplings of cardiac muscles, and we think that it is at these sites that the action potential traveling along the surface membrane triggers the release of calcium from the junctional sarcoplasmic reticulum (10,11).

As illustrated in electron micrographs of portal vein and main pulmonary artery, there are different amounts of sarcoplasmic reticulum in different smooth muscles. Semiquantitative electron

microscopy shows that there is a significant difference between the
fraction of cell volume occupied by the sarcoplasmic reticulum in
the pulmonary artery and the aorta on the one hand, and in the portal vein, mesenteric artery and taenia coli on the other (11). The
smooth muscle of the large arteries has a much larger volume of
sarcoplasmic reticulum than do the other smooth muscles. The estro-
gen treated uterus also has a rather large volume of sarcoplasmic
reticulum, also suggesting that a well developed sarcoplasmic reticulum is correlated with the protein-synthetic functions of smooth
muscles.

There is a correlation between the volume of the sarcoplasmic
reticulum and the behavior of the different smooth muscles. The
smooth muscles that have a larger volume of sarcoplasmic reticulum
can also contract in the absence of extracellular calcium, while
the smooth muscles that contain a very small amount of sarcoplasmic
reticulum either do not contract or contract only minimally (11).
The correlation is so good that one worries about it being fortui-
tous.

Smooth muscles containing a well developed sarcoplasmic reticulum can also be contracted by drugs even if depolarized with high
potassium solutions in the absence of extracellular calcium. Furthermore, the maximal contractions produced by the two different
drugs under such conditions are still unequal. Such experiments
raise the important question of how drugs can release intracellular
stored calcium in the absence of either an increased calcium influx
or depolarization of the already depolarized surface membrane.

Divalent cations can be accumulated by the sarcoplasmic reticulum of smooth muscles in situ. Strontium has a higher atomic
number (38) than calcium (20) and is therefore more electron opaque.
Strontium can also substitute for calcium in a number of physiological processes, including activation of contraction and uptake by
fragmented sarcoplasmic reticulum isolated from striated muscle.

Electron opaque deposits of strontium are found in the sarcoplasmic reticulum of smooth muscles incubated in strontium-containing

Krebs' solution prior to fixation, indicating that the sarcoplasmic
reticulum in smooth muscle can indeed accumulate divalent cations
(14). In addition to the sarcoplasmic reticulum, mitochondria also
contain deposits in vascular and uterine smooth muscles loaded with
strontium prior to fixation.

Energy-dispersive X-ray microanalysis allows us to determine
rigorously the chemical composition of electron opaque deposits,
and to exclude the possibility that they represent osmiophilic
structures rather than specific cation deposits. The characteristic X-ray photons emitted as the deposits are irradiated with
electron beams of sufficiently high intensity to show that in smooth
muscles incubated with strontium, the mitochondria-containing
granules emit a K_a peak at 14.2 KeV characteristic of the strontium
emission. Calcium (K_a) peaks have also been detected over such
mitochondria (15).

Such observations suggest, but do not prove, the possibility
that mitochondria may play a role in the regulation of cytoplasmic
calcium levels in smooth muscle.

Finally, we should define the mechanism of the contractile process, activated by calcium, in smooth muscle. For some 15 years of
electron microscopic studies several laboratories have been unable
to demonstrate consistently thick filaments as the organized form
of myosin in vertebrate smooth muscles. Therefore, the question
of whether a sliding filament mechanism operates in smooth muscle
was left unsettled.

More recent studies, using improved techniques of fixation,
demonstrated thick filaments in vascular, intestinal, uterine and
vas deferens smooth muscle. The presence of these filaments is
independent of the contractile state of the muscle. In rabbit portal vein the thick (myosin) filaments are approximately 155 Å in
diameter. Surrounding them, sometimes forming rosettes, is a
second set of (actin) filaments 50 to 80 Å in diameter. The best
preserved preparations show a fairly regular side-to-side lattice
of thick and thin filaments (5,16,17).

In striated muscle the contractile mechanism is mediated by
crossbridges on the thick filaments, and the question arises as to
whether there are such crossbridges on the thick filaments in
smooth muscle. On suitable ultra-thin sections of smooth muscle,
there is indeed a suggestion of periodic connections between the
thick and adjacent thin filaments, suggestive of a crossbridge-like
arrangement (5). It is probable, therefore, that calcium in smooth,
as in striated, muscles activates a sliding-filament mechanism of
contraction.

REFERENCES

1. A. P. Somlyo and A. V. Somlyo, Pharmacol. Rev., 22: 249 (1970).

2. A. P. Somlyo, The Physiologist, 15: 338 (1972).

3. A. P. Somlyo, A. V. Somlyo, and V. Smiesko, Advan. Cyclic
    Nucleotide Res., 1: 175 (1972).

4. R. M. Bagby, A. M. Young, R. S. Dotson, A. B. Fisher, and
    K. McKinnon, Nature (London), 234: 351 (1971).

5. A. P. Somlyo, C. E. Devine, A. V. Somlyo, and R. V. Rice,
    Phil. Trans. Roy. Soc. London, B 265: 223 (1973).

6. A. V. Somlyo and A. P. Somlyo, J. Pharmacol. Exp. Ther., 159:
    129 (1968).

7. A. V. Somlyo, P. Vinall, and A. P. Somlyo, Microvasc. Res., 1:
    354 (1969).

8. D. H. L. Evans, H. O. Schild, and S. Thesleff, J. Physiol.
    (London), 143: 474 (1958).

9. A. P. Somlyo and A. V. Somlyo in "Vascular Neuroeffector
    "Systems," eds. J. A. Bevan, R. F. Furchgott, R. A. Maxwell,
    and A. P. Somlyo, S. Karger, Basel, 1971, pp. 216-226.

10. A. P. Somlyo, C. E. Devine, A. V. Somlyo, and S. R. North,
    J. Cell Biol., 51: 722 (1971).

11. C. E. Devine, A. V. Somlyo, and A. P. Somlyo, J. Cell Biol.,
    52: 690 (1972).

12. R. Ross and S. J. Klebanoff, J. Cell Biol., 50: 159 (1971).

13. A. P. Somlyo and A. V. Somlyo, Pharmacol. Rev., 20: 197 (1968).

14. A. V. Somlyo and A. P. Somlyo, Science, 174: 955 (1971).

15. A. P. Somlyo, A. V. Somlyo, C. E. Devine, P. D. Peters, and
    T. A. Hall, J. Cell Biol., 61: 723 (1974).

16. A. P. Somlyo, A. V. Somlyo, C. E. Devine, and R. V. Rice,
     Nature New Biol., 231: 243 (1971).

17. A. W. Jones, A. P. Somlyo, and A. V. Somlyo, J. Physiol.
     (London), 232: 247 (1973).

Chapter 16

CALCIUM EXCHANGE IN THE HEART

Harald Reuter

Department of Pharmacology
University of Bern
Bern, Switzerland

We have heard in the previous talks that calcium is very
important for muscle function. And we have also heard that for
controlling the intracellular Ca concentration in muscle the sarcolemma seems to play an important role. The cardiac muscle is by
no means an exception in this respect. What I want to talk about
is how the movements of Ca ions across the sarcolemma of the
cardiac muscle fibers can be envisaged.

I want to summarize very briefly excitation-contraction
coupling in the heart as I see it (for extensive reviews see 1,2).
During the action potential there is an increase in the Ca permeability of the membrane, which by some unknown mechanism triggers
the release of intracellular Ca and, at least under certain conditions, also contributes directly to the change in the free
cellular Ca ion concentration in the myoplasm. The myoplasmic Ca
ion concentration at rest is very low, namely, on the order of
10^{-7} M. If Ca is released from the sarcoplasmic reticulum the
myoplasmic Ca concentration can increase by approximately two
orders of magnitude. This causes activation of the contractile
system. When Ca is taken up again by the sarcoplasmic reticulum
the muscle relaxes. Ca is probably stored in the flattened end
sacs of the sarcoplasmic reticulum, which are in close proximity

to the sarcolemma not only at the T tubules but also at the
surface membrane.

If the membrane is permeable to Ca ions, without any Ca outward transport system there would be very soon an overload of the
sarcoplasmic reticulum and of the mitochondria with Ca. Such a Ca
outward transport system has to be located in the sarcolemma in
order to be able to reduce the overall intracellular Ca concentration.

In the following discussion the main evidence regarding the
mechanisms of these Ca movements across the sarcolemma of cardiac
cells will be presented.

CALCIUM INWARD MOVEMENT DURING THE CARDIAC ACTION POTENTIAL

The conditions for passive Ca influx in cardiac muscle during
excitation are (1) a large inwardly directed electrochemical
gradient for Ca ions across the sarcolemma, and (2) permeability
changes of the membrane to Ca ions during depolarization.

Tracer methods offer one possibility to measure Ca influx
during excitation (3,4,5). However, the tracer exchange measurements do not indicate during which phase of the cardiac action
potential Ca influx occurs, nor are they able to provide information about the mechanism and the kinetics of Ca influx during
depolarization of the membrane. To answer these questions electrophysiological techniques provide a powerful tool. Intracellular
recordings of cardiac action potentials and particularly voltage-
clamp measurements resolved some of these problems.

During which phase of the cardiac action potential does
calcium influx occur? Figure 1 shows the effects of increasing
the extracellular Ca concentration and of adrenaline on action
potentials of cardiac Purkinje fibers.

In both conditions Ca influx as measured by tracer methods
is increased (3,6,7). If the Ca influx during the action potential
is electrogenic one would expect a depolarization of the cell

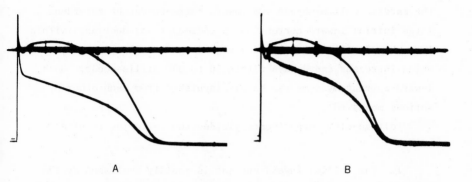

A   B

FIG. 1.   Superimposed action potentials of two Purkinje fibers
(sheep).   (A) Effect of change in [Ca]o from 0.45 mM (lower trace)
to 7.2 mM (upper trace—resting potential is -81 mV.   (B) Control
(lower trace) and effect of adrenaline 5 x 10^{-7} g/ml (upper trace)—
resting potential is -85 mV.   Upstrokes of action potentials have
been retouched.   (From Ref. 9.)

membrane. This can be seen during the plateau phases of the action

potentials in Figure 1. Similar effects have also been demonstra-

ted on action potentials of several other cardiac tissues. Even in

Na-free solution or in the presence of tetrodotoxin, i.e., under

conditions where the inward Na current is abolished, an increase in

extracellular Ca or Sr or the addition of catecholamines can re-

store long-lasting action potentials. On the other hand, the

trivalent and divalent cations La, Mn, Co or Ni, reduce the plateau

phase of cardiac action potentials and abolish the regenerative

responses in Na-free or tetrodotoxin-containing solutions (8).

These experiments provide strong circumstantial evidence that Ca

influx occurs primarily during the plateau phase of the cardiac

action potential.

This evidence is strongly supported by voltage-clamp measure-

ments. The voltage-clamp method permits holding the membrane

potential constant at any level and for any time, while the

currents required to offset the membrane potential are recorded.

These currents are directly proportional to the ionic currents

flowing through the membrane. During stepwise depolarization of

the cardiac cell membrane two inward currents can be recorded: a
large initial inward current which increases and decreases within
less than 5 milliseconds, and a second much smaller inward current
which increases and decays within 50 to 300 milliseconds. Both
inward current systems can be distinguished from each other by
various means (8).

Voltage-clamp experiments yielded the following results:

1. The initial inward current is rapidly abolished by the
removal of external Na, while the slow inward current is very
little affected.

2. The initial inward current is greatly reduced or elimina-
ted by tetrodotoxin, while this poison has no affect on the slow
inward current.

3. The initial inward current is completely "inactivated" by
a long-lasting offset of the membrane potential to about -50 mV,
while the slow inward current is only recorded at potentials above
-50 mV (Fig. 2).

4. The slow inward current is very sensitive to alterations
in the external Ca concentration (Fig. 2), while the effects on the
initial inward current are small and variable. Sr, but not Mg,
can replace Ca in generating the slow inward current.

5. The cations, La, Mn, Co or Ni, and the drugs verapamil
and D 600 (methoxy derivative of verapamil), greatly reduce or
abolish the slow inward current, while the initial inward current
is not much affected. These cations, like Ca or Sr, shift the
conductance variables of the initial inward Na current in the depolarizing direction. However, their action on the slow inward
current is independent of the shift of the Na conductance variables
and is opposite to Ca or Sr.

6. Catecholamines greatly increase the slow inward current,
while they have no effect on the initial inward current. The catecholamine effect on the slow inward current is still present under
conditions of the initial inward current being abolished by

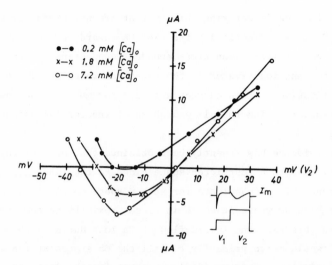

FIG. 2. Current-voltage relations of slow inward current measured in a canine ventricular fiber in Tyrode solution with three
different calcium concentrations (0.2 mM, filled circles; 1.8 mM,
crosses; 7.2 mM, open circles). The first potential step, V_1, was
always from the resting potential (-75 mV) to -44 mV in order to
inactivate I_{Na} at the variable potential step V_2 (inset). Plotted
are maximum inward (negative) or minimum outward current (positive;
ordinate) flowing at the variable potential step V_2 (internal potential; abscissa). (From Ref. 10.)

tetrodotoxin, the continuous depolarization of the membrane po-

tential, or the absence of external Na.

The sensitivity of the rapid initial inward current to varia-

tion in external Na suggests that it is carried by Na ions. The

kinetics of the initial inward Na current cannot be resolved ac-

curately with the presently available methods. However, qualita-

tively it accounts for the rapid depolarization phase of the

cardiac action potential. The slow inward current can be measured

fairly accurately by the voltage-clamp method. The strong depen-

dence of this current on the presence of external Ca and its

insensitivity to external Na suggest that Ca ions are the primary

charge carriers. However, in some cardiac tissues, Na ions seem

to contribute to this current to a variable extent, i.e., the

conductance channels carrying this current are not perfectly selective for Ca ions. Kinetically the slow Ca inward current can be
described as a voltage- and time-dependent conductance system which
is activated and inactivated in the potential range of -50 to +10
mV. Quantitatively, this current accounts for most of the inward
charge transfer during the plateau phase of the cardiac action
potential.

Some evidence has recently been obtained that most of this
current flows into a restricted space close to the inner surface of
the membrane (2). A candidate for such a space could be the sarcoplasmic reticulum where it comes in close proximity to the sarcolemma. In this case the inward flow of Ca ions during each action
potential would serve primarily to fill the Ca stores of the sarcoplasmic reticulum. This would also account for the intimate, but,
at least in mammalian ventricular muscle, indirect relation between
the slow inward Ca current and the activation of contraction (11).
An extensive hypothesis for this relation has been described by
Bassingthwaighte and Reuter (2).

CALCIUM OUTWARD TRANSPORT (Na-Ca EXCHANGE)

As shown in the preceding section, the cardiac cell membrane
is permeable to Ca ions. Since passive Ca movements are inward,
the cell would be overloaded with Ca if there were no outward
transport of this ion. Only recently some features of Ca outward
transport from cardiac muscle have been described (12,13). A very
similar Ca transport system has also been found in squid axon (14,
15) (for reviews see 16). In cardiac muscle the basic features of
Ca outward transport are the following:

1. A large fraction (more than 80%) of Ca efflux is dependent
on the presence of external Na and Ca. Under normal conditions the
bulk of Ca efflux is an exchange with external Na (Na-Ca exchange),
and only a small fraction is an exchange with external Ca (Ca-Ca
exchange).

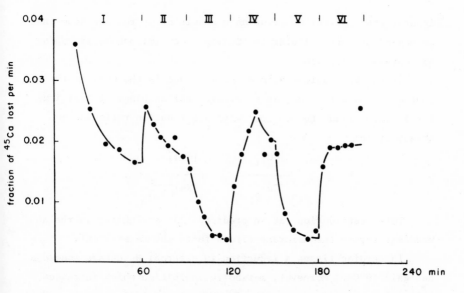

FIG. 3.   Effects of changing $[Ca]_o$ and $[Na]_o$ on ^{45}Ca efflux
from a guinea-pig auricle in the presence and absence of 0.2 mM/1
$LaCl_3$. Abscissa: time of tracer washout in minutes; ordinate:
fraction of ^{45}Ca lost per minute. The roman figures indicate experimental periods with different ion composition of the rinsing
solutions. La was in the solutions during periods I to III.
Period I: Na-containing, Ca-free solution; Periods II, IV, and VI:
Na- and Ca- (1.8 mM/1) containing Tyrode's solution; Periods III
and V: Na- and Ca-free solution in which NaCl was isosmotically
replaced by choline Cl; all solutions were buffered with Tris HCl
to pH 7.2 at 35°C. (From Ref. 17.)

2. Quantitatively, two Na ions and one Ca ion compete for one
transport site (carrier) on both sides of the membrane.

3. The carrier does not have much affinity for K, Li, Mg or
La ions (Fig. 3) while the affinity for Sr is approximately the
same as for Ca.

4. The temperature coefficient (Q_{10}) for Ca efflux between
3° and 35°C is 1.35, which is surprisingly low for an uphill
transport. Furthermore, metabolic inhibitors like 2,4-dinitrophe-
nol or cyanide increase rather than decrease Ca efflux. This may
be due to an increase in the free Ca ion concentration close to the

inner surface of the membrane as a result of Ca release from ener-
gy-dependent intracellular Ca binding sites (mitochondria and/or
sarcoplasmic reticulum).

If the Na gradient across the membrane is the only energy
source for Ca extrusion, an electroneutral exchange of 2 Na ions
for 1 Ca ion leads to the following distribution ratio in the
steady state:

$$\frac{[Ca]_i}{[Ca]_o} = \frac{[Na]_i^2}{[Na]_o^2}$$

This distribution ration predicts that any change in the Na
gradient across the membrane also affects the Ca gradient.

In cardiac tissue a reduction in external Na causes indeed a
net gain in Ca. Moreover, metabolic inhibition which increases
internal Na also increases the Ca content in cardiac muscle. While
these results are in qualitative agreement with such a distribution
ratio, there are quantitative difficulties. The Na gradient $[Na]_i$/
$[Na]_o$ is roughly 1/10, hence the ratio $[Ca]_i/[Ca]_o$ would be 1/100,
i.e., with $[Ca]_o$ 10^{-3}M $[Ca]_i$ would be 10^{-5}M. This concentration
cannot represent the free myoplasmic Ca ion concentration during
relaxation, which must not be much higher than 10^{-7}M. Either there
has to be a Ca compartment close to the membrane where the free Ca
ion concentration is much higher than in the myoplasm (sarcoplasmic
reticulum?) or one has to postulate another energy source in
addition to the Na gradient. At present there is no conclusive
evidence whether or not energy sources other than the Na gradient
are directly involved in this transport mechanism. Indirectly, of
course, ATP breakdown, which is required for Na transport, must be
involved in the maintenance of the Na gradient.

REFERENCES

1. S. Ebashi, M. Endo, and I. Ohtsuki, Quart. Rev. Biophys.,
    2: 351 (1969).

2. J. B. Bassingthwaighte and H. Reuter, in "Electrical phenomena
    in the heart," ed. W.D. De Mello, Academic Press, New York,
    1972, Chap. 13.

3. S. Winegrad and A.M. Shanes, J. Gen. Physiol., 45: 371 (1962).

4. R. Niedergerke, J. Physiol. (London), 167: 551 (1963).

5. G. A. Langer and A. J. Brady, J. Gen. Physiol., 46: 703 (1963).

6. A. Grossman and R. F. Furchgott, J. Pharmacol. Exp. Ther.,
    145: 162 (1964).

7. H. Reuter, Naunyn-Schmiedebergs Arch. Pharmakol., 251: 401
    (1965).

8. H. Reuter, Progr. Biophys. Mol. Biol., 26: 1 (1973).

9. H. Reuter, J. Physiol. (London), 192: 479 (1967).

10. G. W. Beeler, Jr., and H. Reuter, J. Physiol. (London), 207:
    191 (1970).

11. G. W. Beeler, Jr., and H. Reuter, J. Physiol. (London), 207:
    211 (1970).

12. H. Reuter and N. Seitz, J. Physiol (London), 195: 451 (1968).

13. H. G. Glitsch, H. Reuter, and H. Scholz, J. Physiol. (London),
    209: 25 (1970).

14. P. F. Baker, M. P. Blaustein, A. L. Hodgkin, and R. A. Stein-
    hardt, J. Physiol. (London), 200: 431 (1969).

15. M. P. Blaustein and A. L. Hodgkin, J. Physiol. (London), 200:
    497 (1969).

16. P. F. Baker, Progr. Biophys. Mol. Biol., 24: 177 (1972).

17. B. G. Katsung, H. Reuter, and H. Porzig, Experientia, 29:1073
    (1973).

CHAPTER 17

CHEMISTRY OF THE PROSTAGLANDINS

John E. Pike

The Upjohn Company
Kalamazoo, Michigan

I think in a very real sense the explosion of the prostaglandin literature began with the structure elucidation and the knowledge that these materials were novel in a chemical sense (1).
The structures of the two currently most interesting prostaglandins, prostaglandin E_2 and prostaglandin $F_{2\alpha}$, are shown in
Figure 1. Before describing a series of structures I think perhaps
it's worth trying to define what prostaglandins are. Prostaglandins are a family of naturally occurring fatty acids. Perhaps I
could expand a little on that definition. I think it's important
to emphasize the fact that this is a family of compounds. We are
not talking about one compound, one structure, or two structures,

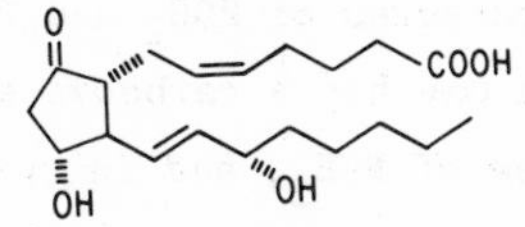

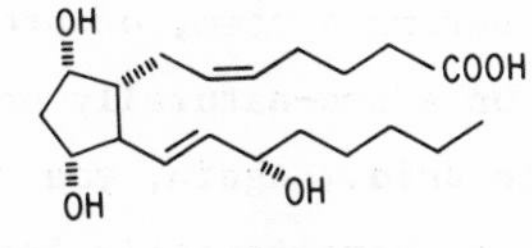

PGE$_2$

PGF$_{2\alpha}$

FIG. 1. Structures of PGE$_2$ and PGF$_{2\alpha}$

183

but about a family of compounds that are all very closely related
chemically, with very small structural variations. These small
structural variations are associated with quite different biological properties. Secondly, of course, they are naturally occurring,
and I think that's self-explanatory. They are found in most
mammals and, of course, in man. Again, they are fatty acids. Perhaps this is extending the definition of what people normally
think of as fatty acids. Depending upon what one's discipline is,
one thinks of fatty acids in different ways. Chemists, taking my
own case, think of fatty acids as a rather uninteresting series of
long-chain carbon compounds terminating in a carboxyl, with what
seems a rather inexplicable distribution of double bonds along the
carbon chain. In calling prostaglandins fatty acids one has to
realize that they are somewhat unique members of the group. They
still have a carboxyl at the terminal position, but they're very
different in that they have undergone enzymatic changes involving
the formation of a five-membered ring and have incorporated three
oxygen atoms. The incorporation of oxygen causes a lot of changes
in the properties of the molecule. For example, they become a lot
more aqueous soluble than the typical fatty acids. Of course
they're associated with a very different spectrum of biological
activity compared to the simple long-chain saturated or unsaturated
fatty acids.

The only way the structures of PGE_2 and $PGF_{2\alpha}$ differ is that
on the five-membered ring one has a carbonyl group, a ketone in
this position, in the case of PGE_2, and in the case of $PGF_{2\alpha}$ one
has a hydroxyl group. We can look at prostaglandin structures in a
little more detail (Fig. 2), and I think it is necessary to define
the nomenclature, the numbering system, of prostaglandins. The
prostaglandins are based on a non-naturally occurring parent skeletal acid called prostanoic acid. Again, you see the five-membered
ring which is, of course, a characteristic feature of prostaglandins. There are two side chains, one a carboxy side chain, and
the lower an alkyl side chain. The numbering system, as with

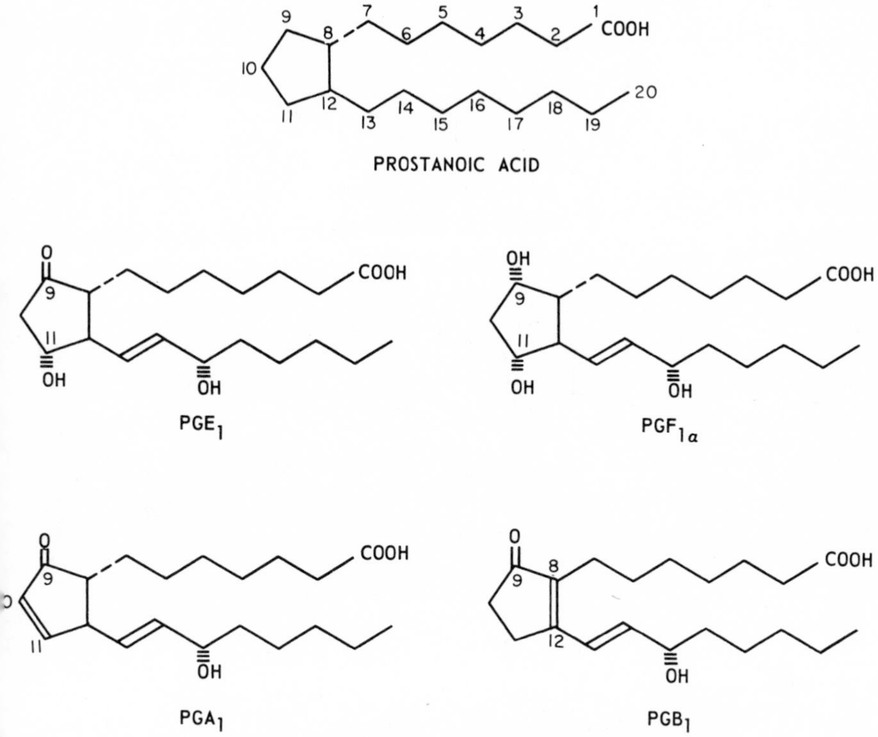

PROSTANOIC ACID

PGE₁   PGF₁ₐ

PGA₁   PGB₁

FIG. 2.   Prostaglandin structures.

typical fatty acids, starts with the carbon of the carboxyl, then
goes down the chain toward the five-membered ring. Numbering con-
tinues around the ring and then through the lower side chain to the
C-20 carbon. The prostaglandins are described by both number and
letter. In this table we show the nomenclature by letter in the
1 series. PGE₁ and PFG₁ₐ were the two prostaglandins first characterized by Bergström and Sjovall. One sees the characteristic
features—the five-membered ring, 9 carbonyl, 9 hydroxyl, the
other oxygen atom on the five-membered ring in the 11 position,
double bond in the 13,14 position, and a very important feature—
the 15 hydroxyl. Thus, the E compounds have a carbonyl, the F
compounds have a hydroxyl. The A compounds are formed by a

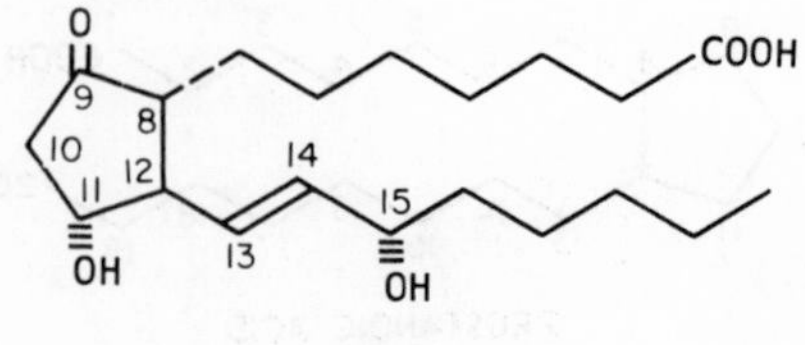

FIG. 3.   Examples of the prostaglandin numbering system.

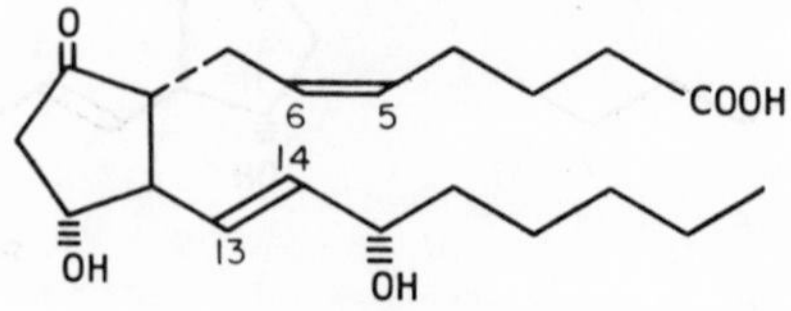

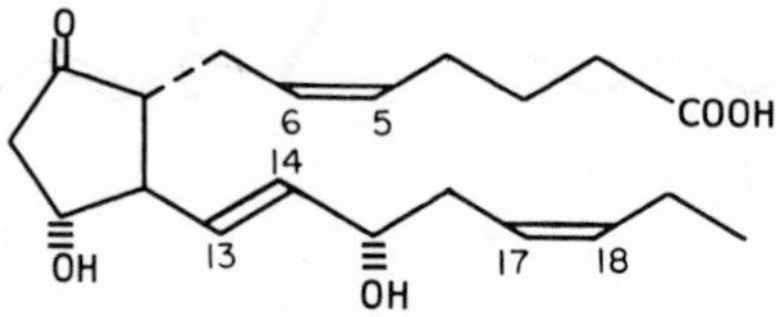

dehydration of the β-hydroxy ketone system of the E compound to give an unsaturated ketone with a double bond at the 10, 11 position, and still a carbonyl at position 9--for example, PGA_1. Of course, there are comparable A compounds in the 2 and 3 series. If one treats the A compounds with base, one can obtain an isomer of this compound with the double bond now moved to the 8, 12 position, PGB_1.

In Figure 3 we see the significance of the numbering system—what we mean when we say E_1, as opposed to E_2 or E_3. A simple way perhaps, of remembering this is that E_1 has one double bond in the 13, 14 position; E_2 has two double bonds, a 13, 14 double bond

which is a trans double bond, and a 5, 6 double bond which is a cis
double bond. PGE_3 has three double bonds, and compared to PGE_2
has an additional cis double bond at the 17, 18 position.

It is important to emphasize in a little more detail the importance of the stereochemistry of prostaglandins, and to appre-
ciate the critical nature of the arrangement of the different substituents in stereochemical terms. I think the best analogy one
can think of is the steroids, where again the stereochemistry of
perhydrophenanthrene system, and of the functional groups are, of
course, very important. One way of starting to think about the
stereochemistry is, for example, to look at $PGF_{1\alpha}$. In the first
instance, the simplest generalization is to think of the five-
numbered ring as essentially flat. This is not strictly true, but
to get some fix on understanding stereochemistry I think this is a
good way to begin. The carboxy side chain is oriented below the
plane of the five-membered ring. In other words, we would call it
α oriented by analogy with the steroid numbering system. The alkyl
side chain is then oriented above the plane of the five-membered
ring. Bearing that in mind, one can then define or name the substituents on the five-membered ring (two hydroxyl groups at 9 and
11) as, again, α oriented. α indicates a position below the plane
of the five-membered ring, while β oriented would be above the
plane of the five-membered ring. So both the hydroxyl groups in
$PGF_{1\alpha}$ are on the same side of the five-membered ring as the carboxy
side chain and, therefore, are α oriented.

If one chemically reduces the carbonyl group of PGE_1, one gets
two hydroxyl isomers at C-9. One, the natural compound, $PGF_{1\alpha}$; the
other the epimer $PGF_{1\beta}$, which differs only from $PGF_{1\alpha}$ in that this
hydroxyl group is now β oriented, or above the plane of the five-
membered ring. Another very important aspect is the nomenclature
of the C-15 position. This is a very critical part of the molecule
and here the stereochemistry of this can be defined in two ways.
It can again be defined in terms of the α and β nomenclature,
so that the natural configuration would be 15 α-hydroxyl.

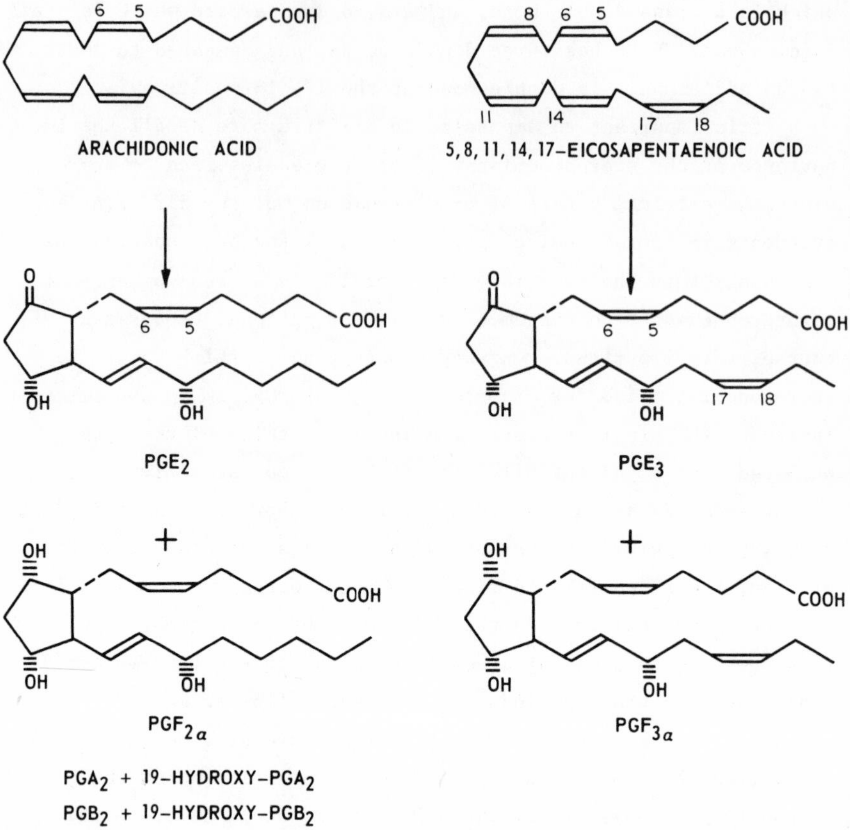

6 5
COOH
ARACHIDONIC ACID
8 6 5
COOH
11 14 17 18
5,8,11,14,17-EICOSAPENTAENOIC ACID
O
6 5
COOH
OH
OH
PGE2
O
6 5
COOH
OH
OH
17 18
PGE3
+
OH
COOH
OH
OH
PGF2a
+
OH
COOH
OH
OH
PGF3a
PGA2 + 19-HYDROXY-PGA2
PGB2 + 19-HYDROXY-PGB2

FIG. 4. Formation of prostaglandins.

Unfortunately, chemists don't always agree on nomenclature systems, so you'll find in the literature this stereochemistry defined in many different ways. For example, in some work it's been called 15S. I think the most correct type of nomenclature is to define the chirality of this center, the stereochemistry of this carbon atom, in an SR system. So, in fact, if one calls the 15α the normal configuration of the natural product that is also 15S. If one inverts the hydroxyl and the hydrogen of this position, the hydroxyl would then be 15β oriented, or in 15R configuration. The configuration of this center is very critical for biological

activity. Natural compounds are usually 15S, the isomers there
are 15R.

Perhaps that's enough of the grammar, as it were, of the
prostaglandins. Figure 4 shows how these compounds are formed.
Again, we have similar routes to give PGE_2 and $PGF_{2\alpha}$ and PGE_3 and
$PGF_{2\alpha}$. It has been well established originally by Samuelsson
working in Bergström's group, and VanDorp, that arachidonic acid is
the enzymatic or biosynthetic precursor of the 2 series of prostaglandins (2). What occurs is a cyclization to form a five-membered
ring and incorporation of three oxygen atoms. So arachidonic acid
leads to PGE_2 and $PGF_{2\alpha}$, and the corresponding fatty acid with
five double bonds is a precursor of PGE_3 and $PGF_{3\alpha}$, and bis-
homo-γ-linolenic acid is the precursor of PGE_1 and $PGF_{1\alpha}$.

Figure 5 shows that these polyunsaturated fatty acids are
derived originally from phospholipids by the action of a phospholipase and that the free polyunsaturated fatty acid serves as a
substrate for the prostaglandin synthesis complex of enzymes. This
is then, of course, converted as shown on the earlier slide to PGE_2.

One very interesting feature of the biosynthesis is that both
the oxygen atoms that end up on the 9 and 11 positions come from
the same oxygen molecule. The fairly well accepted concept of this
mechanism is that an intermediate in this biosynthesis is an
endoperoxide, which goes either to the E or to the F series of
prostaglandins.

For many years we had to rely on a scale-up of this biosynthesis for a source of prostaglandins. The various chemical
methods that I'll mention briefly had not yet been developed. By
incubating, on a relatively large scale, arachidonic acid or the
corresponding bis-homo-γ-linolenic acid with a crude enzyme preparation from the seminal vesicular gland of the sheep, it was
possible to obtain E_2 and $F_{2\alpha}$ and E_1 and $F_{1\alpha}$ (3). And this source,
for many years, served to make these compounds available for a
variety of different studies.

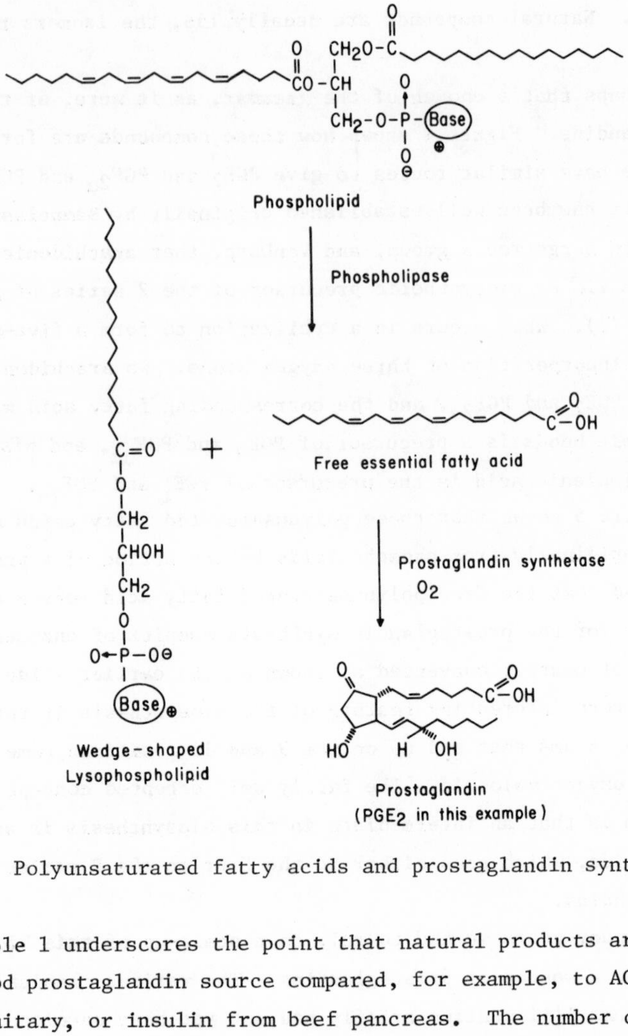

FIG. 5. Polyunsaturated fatty acids and prostaglandin synthesis.

Table 1 underscores the point that natural products are not a
very good prostaglandin source compared, for example, to ACTH from
hog pituitary, or insulin from beef pancreas. The number of human
doses one can obtain per kilogram of the original natural product
is shown in the case of ACTH to be 4000, for insulin 100, and for
$PGF_{2\alpha}$ from sheep glands less than 5, based on the labor-induction
dose.

Following the biosynthesis, there were many different chemical
total syntheses developed (4,5,6). We developed several at Upjohn;
Corey, at Harvard, developed many; and total synthesis is now the

TABLE 1

Yields of Hormones from Natural Sources

Hormone	Source	Human Doses/Kg
ACTH	Hog Pituitaries	4,000-5,000
Insulin	Beef Pancreas	100 - 200
$PGF_{2\alpha}$	Sheep Vesicular Glands	1/5 to 5[a]

[a] for labor induction

best method for making prostaglandins, since one has a degree of
flexibility that enables one to make analogs. The only disadvantage, perhaps, is the relatively large number of distinct chemical
operations necessary to build up the final molecule. One of the
difficulties, as I explained, is the necessity to obtain the right
stereoisomer. In the case of $PGF_{2\alpha}$, for example, there are five
asymmetric centers, and six different functional entities; so this
is a considerable challenge to the organic chemist. I don't think
we need to go into the details of the various routes except to
emphasize that chemical total synthesis is now the way to obtain
the prostaglandins which for many years depended on scale-up
biosynthesis. But in 1969, Weinheimer and Spraggins, at the
University of Oklahoma, reported the isolation of several prostaglandins from a gorgonian, or seawhip, called Plexaura homomalla
(7).

Figure 6 shows the two prostaglandins that they described in
1969. These were PGA compounds. The source was relatively remark-
able by natural-product standards. They obtained between a 1 to 2%
yield of these A prostaglandin isomers from the air-dried cortex
of the gorgonian. There are three different features I'd just like
to draw your attention to here. One is the fact that the methyl
ester was isolated, not the free acid; another point is that the
15 hydroxyl is acetylated and is not a free hydroxyl; and the
third, and perhaps most surprising feature, was that this

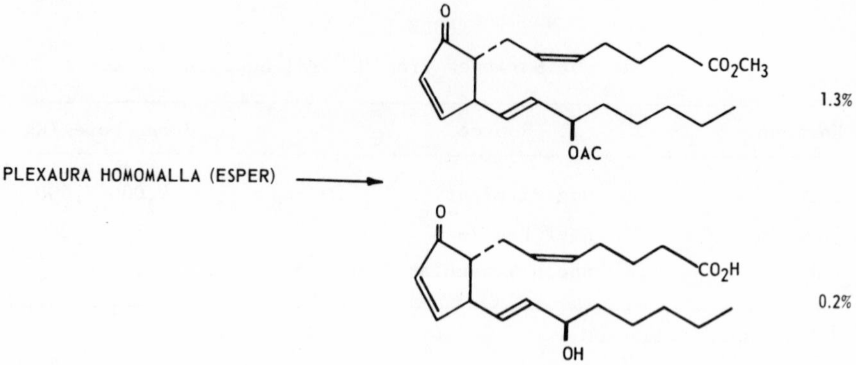

FIG. 6.   Nonmammalian PG source.

15 hydroxyl has the unnatural, epi-, or R, configuration. This
created something of a problem when we tried converting these particular natural products into the mammalian PGE_2 and $PGF_{2\alpha}$. We
were able to effect the change (8), but as a source, the unnatural
stereochemistry at C-15 was, of course, a distinct disadvantage.
For reasons that are rather complex to explain now, we decided to
look at different areas of the Caribbean for this particular
gorgonian, and quite dramatically we found that if one harvested
this very readily available seawhip in other locations, one could
obtain, not the 15R, but the natural 15S prostaglandins (9).

Figure 7 depicts the S coral-derived prostaglandins which
could be obtained from other areas of the Caribbean. Of course,
this made _Plexaura_ _homomalla_ a very much better source. We didn't
have to invert stereochemistry now to get to the mammalian structures, and it was a relatively simple chemical task to convert the
A compounds to the E or the F compounds. It is still quite a
mystery as to why there should be this variation in the stereochemistry at 15 in different locations. In some locations, for
example, one gets almost equal mixtures of the R and S isomers at
C-15.

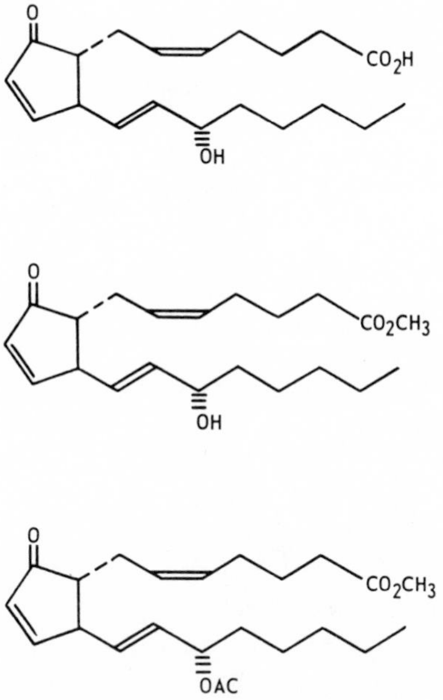

PGA₂

PGA₂ METHYL ESTER

PGA₂, 15-ACETATE, METHYL ESTER

FIG. 7. [S]- coral derived prostaglandins.

Figure 8 indicates how Drs. Bundy and Schneider at Upjohn worked out a conversion of the PGA_2 to PGE_2. This can now be done in perhaps three or four relatively simple operations (10,11). So this makes the Plexaura homomalla a starting material that is relatively easily converted into the mammalian compound. One simply protects the C-15 position as a trimethylsilyl ether, epoxidizes the unsaturated carbonyl with base and hydrogen peroxide, and reduces the epoxy ketone. One obtains two isomers which can be separated later. Reduction with aluminum amalgam gives PGE_2 in a very high overall yield from the starting PGA_2.

Currently, as I explained, total synthesis is still the method of choice for making prostaglandins, but this natural source has provided quite substantial amounts of the naturally-occurring prostaglandins. It's important to emphasize that, in using a raw

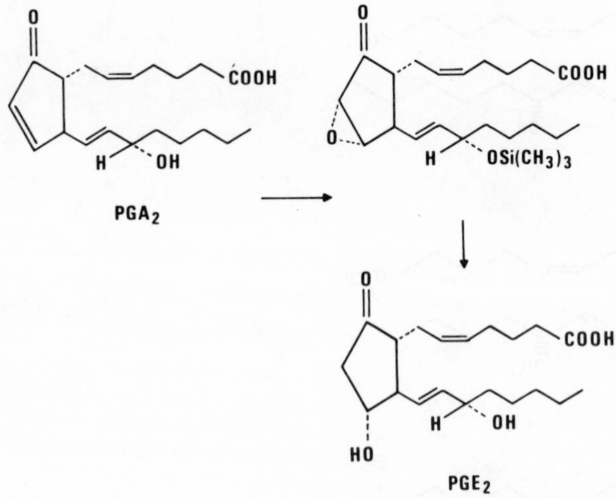

PGA₂

$\longrightarrow$

PGE₂

FIG. 8.   Conversion of PGA$_2$ to PGE$_2$

material like this to make these compounds, one has to be very conscious of ecological considerations.   Just over a year ago we had a
meeting at the Rosensteil School of Marine Sciences, where we presented the controls and the conditions under which we harvested the
coral to the marine scientists, to assure them that this was being
done properly—with concern for regrowth and the balance of the
natural environment (12).

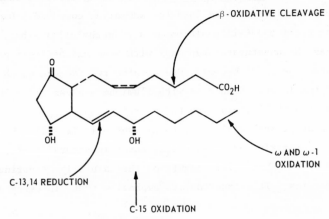

FIG. 9.   Metabolic degradation of prostaglandins.

Figure 9 briefly outlines the metabolic degradation of the
prostaglandins, which has been worked out in great detail in animals and in man, particularly by Samuelsson in Sweden (13). The
first step of this degradation is the oxidation of the 15S hydroxyl
to the corresponding ketone. This enzymatic oxidation is associated with a lowering of some of the biological activities. In other
words, the corresponding 15-keto compounds don't possess all of
the properties of the parent hydroxy compound.

If one wants to make compounds which will not be very rapidly
metabolized, as are the parent prostaglandins, one can introduce
a methyl group at the 15 position (Fig. 10) (8,14,15). This compound should no longer be a substrate for the 15-hydroxy dehydrogenase because there is no way of oxidizing a tertiary hydroxy
compound to the corresponding carbonyl without breaking a carbon-
to-carbon bond, and that is not considered a very likely step. So
by introducing a methyl group here, one has already obtained a very
different series of compounds pharmacologically, and these have
already been evaluated (16,17,18,19,20), both in the area of
obstetrics and gynecology in Sweden and in Uganda, and also as
agents affecting gastric secretion. There are, of course, other
ways of trying to prevent this oxidation from occurring. Another
way we have described is to introduce alkyl groups at the C-16

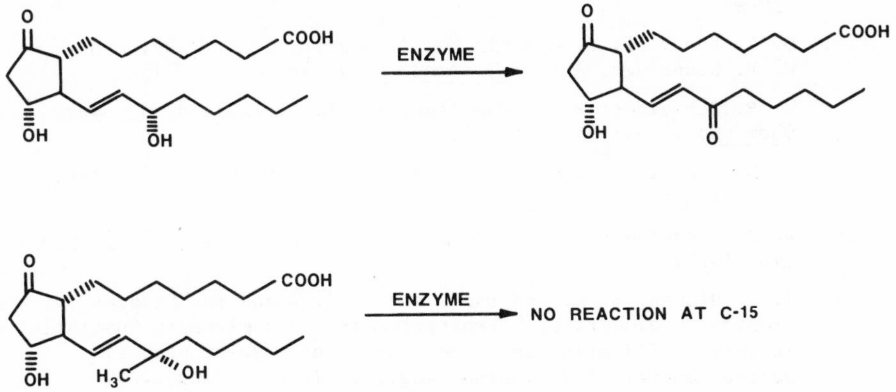

FIG. 10.   Retardation of degradation by 15-position methyl group.

position (21,22). The 16,16-dimethyl compounds have been described
(23). I think one will see quite a lot of prostaglandin analogs;
compounds in which the structures have been varied. These 15-
methyl compounds are just one example of a variety of prostaglandins which we think may have interesting pharmacological activity.

Again, I'd just like to reemphasize the significance of the
stereochemistry, principally because both isomers of the 15-methyl
compounds have been tested clinically. Both the 15S-methyl compounds and the 15R-methyl compounds have interesting biological
properties.

REFERENCES

1. S. Bergström, Science, 157: 382 (1967).

2. B. Samuelsson, Progr. Biochem. Pharmacol., 5: 109 (1969).

3. E. G. Daniels and J. E. Pike, in "Prostaglandin symposium of
   the Worcester foundation for experimental biology, eds. P. W.
   Ramwell and J. E. Shaw, Interscience, New York (1968), p. 379.

4. J. E. Pike, Fortschr. Chem. Org. Naturst., 28: 313 (1970).

5. U. F. Axen, J. E. Pike, and W. P. Schneider in "Progress in
   the total synthesis of natural products," J. W. ApSimon, ed.,
   John Wiley and Sons, 1973.

6. N. M. Weinshenker and N. H. Andersen in "The prostaglandins,"
   vol. 1, ed. P. W. Ramwell, Plenum Press, N.Y., 1973.

7. A. J. Weinheimer and R. L. Spraggins, Tetrahedron Lett., 5185
   (1969).

8. G. L. Bundy, F. H. Lincoln, N. A. Nelson, J. E. Pike, and
   W. P. Schneider, Ann. N.Y. Acad. Sci., 180: 76 (1971).

9. W. P. Schneider, R. D. Hamilton, and L. E. Rhuland, J. Amer.
   Chem. Soc., 94: 2122 (1972).

10. G. L. Bundy, W. P. Schneider, F. H. Lincoln, and J. E. Pike,
    J. Amer. Chem. Soc., 94: 2123 (1972).

11. W. P. Schneider, G. L. Bundy, and F. H. Lincoln, Chem. Commun.,
    254 (1973).

12. J. W. Hinman, S. R. Anderson, and M. H. Simon in "Studies in
    tropical oceanography," Prostaglandins from plexaura homomalla:
    ecology, utilization and conservation of a major medical
    marine source. A Symposium, eds., F. M. Bayer and A. J.
    Weinheimer, University of Miami Press, 1974.

13. B. Samuelsson, E. Granström, K. Green, and M. Hamberg, Ann.
    N.Y. Acad. Sci., 180: 138 (1971).

14. E. W. Yankee and G. L. Bundy, J. Amer. Chem. Soc., 94: 3651
    (1972).

15. G. L. Bundy, E. W. Yankee, J. R. Weeks, and W. L. Miller in
    "Advances in the biosciences 9," Pergamon Press, Vieweg, 1973,
    p. 125.

16. A. Robert and B. J. Magerlein in "Advances in the biosciences
    9," Pergamon Press, Vieweg, 1973, p. 247.

17. S. M. M. Karim, D. C. Carter, D. Bhana, and P. Adaikan
    Ganesan in "Advances in the biosciences 9," Pergamon Press,
    Vieweg, 1973, p. 255.

18. S. M. M. Karim, D. C. Carter, D. Bhana, and A. P. Ganesan,
    Brit. Med. J., 1: 143 (1973).

19. S. M. M. Karim and S. D. Sharma, J. Obstet. Gynaecol. Br.
    Commonw., 79: 737 (1972).

20. M. Bygdeman, F. Beguin, M. Toppozada, and N. Wiqvist in
    "The prostaglandins: clinical applications in human repro-
    duction," ed., E. M. Southern, Futura, Mount Kisco, New York,
    1972.

21. B. J. Magerlein, D. W. DuCharme, W. E. Magee, W. L. Miller,
    A. Robert, and J. R. Weeks, Prostaglandins, 4: 143 (1973).

22. M. Hayashi, H. Miyake, T. Tanouchi, S. Iguchi, Y. Ighchi,
    and F. Tanouchi, J. Org. Chem., 38: 1250 (1973).

23. S. M. M. Karim, D. C. Carter, D. Bhana, and P. A. Ganesan,
    Int. Res. Commun. Syst. (73-3) 8-3-2 (1973).

CHAPTER 18

PROSTAGLANDINS AND CYCLIC AMP

John M. Marsh
University of Miami School of Medicine
Miami, Florida

I am going to discuss some studies done by our laboratory and by others, which have demonstrated an interaction of prostaglandins and cyclic AMP. It was suspected some time ago by investigators such as Ramwell and Shaw (1), that cyclic AMP might be involved in some prostaglandin actions, since in most tissues where prostaglandins produced effects cyclic AMP had been shown to be involved in some hormonal process. A large number of studies on different tissues have now been carried out, and it appears that most of the effects of prostaglandins on cyclic-AMP-mediated processes can be classified as one of two general types.

In the first type, it is believed that prostaglandins are involved in a negative-feedback loop. Cyclic AMP is increased by hormonal action and in turn gives rise to an increased synthesis or release of prostaglandins. The prostaglandins then reduce the concentration of cyclic AMP by either interfering with hormonal stimulation of adenyl cyclase or by stimulating the phosphodiesterase enzyme which destroys cyclic AMP. In the second type, it is believed that prostaglandins act in some way as an intermediate in the action of the hormone on the adenyl cyclase enzyme system.

The first type of effect can be illustrated by the studies

This paper was prepared for, and presented at, the Second Annual Clinical Pharmacology Symposium, University of Miami School of Medicine, March, 1973.

199

carried out on the role of prostaglandin in the hormonal stimulation of lipolysis in adipose tissue. It is well known that many
hormones, including epinephrine, norepinephrine, glucagon, ACTH,
TSH and others, produce a mobilization of the stored triglyceride
in fat cells by first stimulating the adenyl-cyclase enzyme system
which increases the concentration of endogenous cyclic AMP (2).
Cyclic AMP then activates a protein kinase enzyme which converts an
inactive form of a lipase enzyme to its active form. The activated
lipase enzyme then catalyzes the breakdown of triglyceride to
diglyceride and free fatty acid. The diglyceride is then degraded
further; finally, to glycerol and more free fatty acids (3).

Steinberg and coworkers (4) were the first to implicate prostaglandins in this mechanism. They found that if they added Prostaglandin E_1 to incubating rat epididymal fat pads they produced a
rather marked decrease in the lipolysis caused by several hormones.
Butcher and Baird (5) followed up this work and found, using isolated fat cells, that Prostaglandin E_1 also inhibited the hormonal
stimulation of cyclic-AMP accumulation and concluded that the
decreased lipolysis caused by prostaglandins was due to this
lowered level of cyclic AMP.

The mechanism by which prostaglandins inhibit the hormonal
stimulation of cyclic AMP is not clearly understood. There is
evidence which indicates that they act by inhibiting the adenyl
cyclase (6), but there is also some evidence which suggests that
they might stimulate the phosphodiesterase enzyme (7).

It is also believed that endogenous prostaglandins play a
physiological negative-feedback role in this system, for it was
shown by Shaw and Ramwell (8), that hormones which stimulate
lipolysis also stimulate the release of prostaglandins from adipose
tissue in vitro. And finally, in a recent study by Illiano and
Cuatrecasas (9), it was demonstrated that inhibitors of prostaglandin action would enhance the effects of hormones on adipose tissue.
Indomethacin was used as the inhibitor of prostaglandin synthesis,
and 7-oxa-13-prostynoic acid and the compound SC 19220 (a dibenzoxazepine hydrazide) were used as the inhibitors of prostaglandin

effects.   All three agents significantly enhanced the effect of
epinephrine on lipolysis.

A number of different studies could be used to illustrate the
second type of effect of prostaglandins, namely, the role of these
substances as mediators of the hormonal stimulation of adenyl
cyclase.   I have elected, however, to confine most of my remarks on
this topic to our own investigations on the possible role of prostaglandins in the control of steroidogenesis in the corpus luteum
by gonadotropins.

For several years, our laboratory has studied the process of
progesterone synthesis in the corpus luteum and its control by
gonadotropins.   Our approach was to develop an in vitro model
system, where slices of bovine or human corpora lutea were incubated in Krebs-Ringer bicarbonate buffer, and the amounts of progesterone produced were measured.   We found that Luteinizing
Hormone (LH) produced a marked increase in steroidogenesis when it
was added to the incubation and this effect was quite specific for
LH and very sensitive to small amounts of hormone (10).

In our investigation of the mechanism of LH action, we showed
that cyclic AMP was a mediator of this effect, in that LH increased
the endogenous concentration of this cyclic nucleotide (11), and
exogenous cyclic AMP mimicked the effect of the hormone on progesterone synthesis (12).   We have also shown that LH brings about the
increase in endogenous cyclic AMP in the corpus luteum cell by
activating the enzyme, adenyl cyclase (13).

Speroff and Ramwell (14), using this in vitro model system,
then found that exogenous prostaglandins also increased steroidogenesis when added to the incubating slices of bovine corpora lutea.
We attempted then to determine if this stimulation of steroidogenesis by prostaglandins was also mediated by cyclic AMP.   Specifically, we assessed the effect of prostaglandins on the adenyl-
cyclase enzyme system of the homogenates of bovine corpora lutea.
In addition, we attempted to determine if a prostaglandin could be

a mediator of LH, acting between this gonadotropin and its action
on adenyl cyclase.

We found that when Prostaglandin E_2 was added at a concentration of 10 µg/ml to incubating corpora luteal homogenates, there
was a significant increase in adenyl cyclase activity. This increase was only slightly less than that produced by a saturating
concentration of luteinizing hormone (15). In three experiments,
tissue slices were also prepared from the corpora lutea, and the
effect of Prostaglandin E_2 was assessed on progesterone synthesis.
The results confirmed the previous report that Prostaglandin E_2
stimulated steroidogenesis in corpora lutea, and also indicated
that the extent of stimulation of steroidogenesis correlated well
with the increase in adenyl cyclase activity.

The stimulatory effect of prostaglandins on progesterone
synthesis in incubating slices of corpora lutea did appear to be
mediated by cyclic AMP. The second question we then asked was
what the functional significance was of the effect of prostaglandins on adenyl cyclase. We considered the possibility that they
might represent a mediator of the action of LH, acting between LH
and its effect on adenyl cyclase. LH could presumably increase the
concentration of a hypothetical endogenous prostaglandin, which in
turn would stimulate adenyl cyclase. To test this possibility, we
carried out another additive experiment, this time on adenyl
cyclase. The maximal-effective concentration of Prostaglandin E_2
was determined in an homogenate and found to be 100 µg/ml (as shown
by the fact that 1000 µg/ml of Prostaglandin E_2 did not increase
the adenyl cyclase activity over that produced by 100 µg/ml).
Luteinizing hormone was then added with this saturating concentration of prostaglandin to another aliquot of the homogenate. If the
effect of luteinizing hormone was mediated through Prostaglandin E_2,
one would not expect this hormone to increase the activity of the
enzyme in the presence of an already saturating concentration of
prostaglandin. It was found that LH produced a clearly additive
stimulation in addition to the effect of Prostaglandin E_2,

indicating that the two effects are separate phenomena and that
prostaglandins are probably not mediators of the effect of LH (16).

While we were working on these experiments, another group,
headed by Dr. Kuehl of the Merck Institute, was carrying out
similar experiments but came to quite different conclusions (17).
The experimental technique they used was to incubate. whole mouse
ovaries in the presence of ^{14}C-labelled adenine and assess the
effects of LH, PGE_1, and E_2 on the accumulation of ^{14}C-labelled
cyclic AMP. They found, as we had, that LH and the prostaglandins
would increase the cyclic AMP in these tissues. They also considered the possibility that a prostaglandin might be a mediator of
its action on adenyl cyclase, and they tested this possibility
using the prostaglandin antagonist, 7-oxa-13-prostynoic acid. They
found that this antagonist would competatively block the effect of
PGE_1 or E_2, which is expected, since 7-oxa-13-prostynoic acid is a
prostaglandin analogue. They also found, however, that this
inhibitor would competatively block the effect of LH, and they
concluded from these data that a prostaglandin receptor functions
as a necessary intermediate in the action of LH to raise cyclic-AMP
formation (17). Their results were even more intriguing in that
they were also able to demonstrate an additive effect of LH and
prostaglandin. It is very difficult to reconcile the results using
the analogue with the results of both their and our additive
experiments.

We then attempted to carry out experiments such as those
described by Dr. Kuehl, using incubating slices of bovine corpora
lutea, with the difference that we used ^{3}H-labelled adenine instead
of ^{14}C-labelled adenine. Slices of a corpus luteum were incubated
for 1 hour at 37° C in Krebs-Ringer bicarbonate buffer in the
presence of 25 μCi of ⌈^{3}H⌉-adenine. The slices were then rinsed in
isotonic NaCl and incubated again for 30 minutes under control
conditions or in the presence of LH. At the end of the second
incubation, the slices were homogenized, boiled, and centrifuged.
The [^{3}H]-cyclic AMP was isolated from the supernatant by a

TABLE I

Effect of 7-Oxa-13-Prostynoic Acid on [³H]-Cyclic AMP Accumulation in Bovine Corpora Lutea as seen by [³H]-Adenine Incorporation into [³H]-Cyclic AMP (dpm x 10^3/g)

					EXPERIMENTS				
	1	2	3	4	5	6	7	8	9
(1) Control	18	21	135	40	48	31	71	43	267
(2) 1.5 µg/ml LH[a]	440	2110	1840	1180	572	169	4800	1380	3940
(3) 1.5 µg/ml LH + 7-oxa[b]	378	1480	1200	1270	563	115	3410	1590	2420
(4) 0.5 µg/ml LH	232	1060	477	649	229	118	1460	704	1320
(5) 0.5 µg/ml LH + 7-oxa	113	694	472	503	174	54	1350	507	635
(6) 0.15 µg/ml LH	84	436	428	144	189	67	509	550	888
(7) 0.15 µg/ml LH + 7-oxa	73	178	361	192	84	38	397	266	385
(8) 0.05 µg/ml LH	31	114	113	52	51	54	179	101	311
(9) 0.05 µg/ml LH + 7-oxa	16	62	196	47	67	39	127	78	229

[a] LH-NIH-S11

[b] 7-oxa-13-prostynoic acid 50 µg/ml, a gift from Dr. J. Fried of the University of Chicago

modification of the procedure of Krishna et al. (18). The modification involved an additional chromatography of the ^{3}H-labelled
product in a cellulose-thin layer system to achieve radiochemical
purity. Using this technique, we found that LH caused a marked
increase in the accumulation of [^{3}H]-cyclic AMP, which was statistically significant with a p value less than 0.001 and was very
similar in magnitude to the effect we had observed previously on
the accumulation of the mass amounts of cyclic AMP (11).

Nine experiments were carried out in which we assessed the
effect of 7-oxa-13-prostynoic acid on the LH stimulation of
[^{3}H]-cyclic AMP accumulation, and the results are shown in Table I.
LH was added at 4 concentrations (from 0.05 to 1.5 µg/ml) with and
without this analogue (50 µg/ml) to incubating slices of bovine
corpora lutea. As you can see, 7-oxa-13-prostynoic acid did produce an inhibition of the LH effect, but it was not a totally con-
sistent finding. In 5 out of 36 cases the samples treated with the
analogue accumulated more [^{3}H]-cyclic AMP than the samples without
this substance. These values are singled out in Table I by under-
lining the numbers. In addition, we could not demonstrate that
the inhibition we did find was of the competitive type. The
variability of the data was such that we could not construct a
lineweaver-Burk plot through the 7-oxa-13-prostynoic acid points
using a computer program (19).

In summary, I have tried to review some current concepts of
the interaction of prostaglandins and cyclic AMP. In some tissues,
such as the adipose tissue, prostaglandins seem to act as natural
feedback inhibitors modulating the response of the cyclic-AMP
system to hormones. In other tissues, such as the mouse ovary,
there is evidence that prostaglandins may function as an intermediate in the action of hormones on adenyl cyclase. In our model
system, which is the incubated bovine corpus-luteum-slice system,
the situation is still uncertain and awaits further clarification.

REFERENCES

1. P. W. Ramwell and J. E. Shaw, Recent Progr. in Horm. Res., 26: 139 (1970).

2. R. W. Butcher, Pharmacol. Rev., 18: 237 (1966).

3. D. Steinberg and J. K. Huttunen, Advan. Cyclic Nucleotide Res., 1: 47 (1972).

4. D. Steinberg, M. Vaughan, P. J. Nestel, and S. Bergstrom, Biochem. Pharmacol., 12: 764 (1963).

5. R. W. Butcher and C. E. Baird, J. Biol. Chem., 243: 1713 (1968).

6. K. Stock, A. Aulich, and E. Westermann, Life Sci., 7: 113 (1968).

7. R. Paoletti, R. L. Lentati, and Z. Korlkiewicz, "Nobel Symposium 2, Prostaglandins," eds. S. Bergstrom and B. Samuelsson, Almqvist and Weksell, Stockholm, 1967, p. 147.

8. J. E. Shaw and P. W. Ramwell, J. Biol. Chem., 243: 1498 (1968).

9. G. Illiano and P. Cuatrecasas, Nature New Biol., 234: 72 (1971).

10. J. M. Marsh and K. Savard, J. Reprod. and Fert. Suppl., 1: 113 (1966).

11. J. M. Marsh, R. W. Butcher, K. Savard, and E. W. Sutherland, J. Biol. Chem., 241: 5436 (1966).

12. J. M. Marsh and K. Savard, Steroids, 8: 133 (1966).

13. J. M. Marsh, J. Biol. Chem., 245: 1596 (1970).

14. L. Speroff and P. W. Ramwell, J. Clin. Endocrinol., 30: 345 (1970).

15. J. M. Marsh, Fed. Eur. Biochem. Soc., 7: 283 (1970).

16. J. M. Marsh, Ann. N.Y. Acad. Sci., 180: 416 (1971).

17. F. A. Kuehl, Jr., J. L. Humes, J. Tarnoff, V. J. Cirillo, and E. A. Ham, Science, 169: 883 (1970).

18. G. Krishna, B. Weiss, and B. B. Brodie, J. Pharmacol. Exp. Ther., 163: 379 (1968).

19. K. R. Hanson, R. Ling, and E. Havir, Biochem. Biophys. Res. Commun., 29: 194 (1967).

CHAPTER 19

METABOLIC EFFECTS OF PROSTAGLANDINS

Vincent A. Ziboh

Departments of Dermatology and Biochemistry
University of Miami School of Medicine
Miami, Florida

One of the most striking scientific developments in the last
two decades has been the emergence of a group of unsaturated
hydroxy C_{20} carboxylic acids known at prostaglandins. Recent
investigations have established the extraordinary biological significance of these compounds (1,2).

IN VITRO EFFECTS OF PGE_1 ON LIPOLYSIS IN THE ADIPOSE TISSUE

A number of investigators have demonstrated inhibition of
lipolysis in the fat pad with prostaglandins, both in the basal
state and after stimulation by catecholamines and other hormones.

In vitro studies by Steinberg et al. (3,4) on rat adipose
tissue indicated that prostaglandin E_1 (PGE_1) had potent metabolic
effects. It was found that addition of PGE_1 to the incubation
medium lowered the release of glycerol into the incubation medium.
The basal rate from epididymal fat pads of fed rats was inhibited
approximately 30% by 0.1 µg PGE_1/ml of incubation medium. The
studies also showed a dose-dependent inhibition of epinephrine-,
norepinephrine-, glucagon- and ACTH-induced lipolysis by PGE_1. In
another study, PGE_2 was shown to be less potent than PGE_1 in
inhibiting the actions of ACTH and glucagon. No significant difference was shown in the effects of these two prostaglandins on

epinephrine-induced lipolysis. However, in the absence of information on differences in the rates of metabolism of the different
prostaglandins, the significance of these relative differences
cannot truly be evaluated.

Similar observations were confirmed by Bergstrom and Carlson
(5) who reported that glycerol release from human adipose tissue is
suppressed by PGE_1. The release of free fatty acid (FFA) was also
measured in most of these studies. The results generally parallel
closely with those obtained for glycerol. An important exception
encountered in these studies was the effect of PGE_1 in the absence
of lipolytic hormones. In these latter studies, no significant
effect of PGE_1 on basal FFA release was observed even though a
significant suppression of basal glycerol was demonstrated.

These findings have led to the proposal of a hormone-sensitive
triglyceride lipase by Vaughan and Steinberg (6). Although the
enzyme has not been fully purified, the hormone-sensitive triglyceride lipase has been distinguished from that of the more active
monoglyceride lipase (7,8,9,10).

IN VIVO EFFECTS OF PGE_1 ON FAT MOBILIZATION

Intravenous injection of epinephrine 5 μg/kg into anesthetized
dogs caused a marked rise in plasma FFA and blood-glucose levels
(6). When PGE_1 (12.5 μg/kg) is injected simultaneously with
epinephrine, the hyperglycemic action of epinephrine was not
altered but plasma FFA was markedly suppressed. Injection of PGE_1
alone was followed by slight fall in plasma FFA but no definite
change in blood glucose. These results demonstrate the ability of
PGE_1 to suppress mobilization of FFA induced by epinephrine in vivo.
These results are also compatible with those obtained in vitro on
the inhibition of catecholamine lipolysis by PGE_1 in adipose tissue.
There was, however, no apparent effect on the degree of hypergly-
cemia produced by epinephrine. The in vivo effects are, however,
more complex when studied in unstimulated FFA mobilization.

Spellacy et al, (11) found that intravenous infusion of PGE_2 and
$PGF_{2\alpha}$ into pregnant women did not cause a rise in blood glucose or
plasma insulin. The intraveous or intra-aortic infusion of large
doses of PGE_1 lowers FFA in rats (12,13) and in rabbits (14).
However, the intravenous infusion of small doses of PGE_1 (0.2 µg/
kg/minute) into man or dog increases plasma FFA and glycerol (15,16).
These findings suggest that intravenous PGE_1 acts by two independent mechanisms: (1) stimulation via sympathetic-hormone discharge at low dosage as a compensatory reaction to lowered blood
pressure, and (2) inhibition of lipolysis by direct action on the
adipose tissue at high dosage (16,17).

EFFECTS ON GLUCOSE METABOLISM

PGE_1 not only affects the lipolytic process in adipose tissue,
but also influences some aspects of glucose metabolism in a way
similar to insulin.

In isolated rat adipose, PGE_1 stimulates glucose uptake,
glucose oxidation, and triglyceride synthesis (18,19,20).
PGE_1 has also been shown to stimulate, in vitro, glucose
uptake and metabolism in slices of myometrium from pregnant rhesus
monkeys (21). This demonstration of PGE_1 effect on carbohydrate
metabolism in the smooth muscle is unique, since the glycogen level
in the myometrium is directly related to blood-glucose concentration (22).

Skin has been shown to be one of the most active lipid-
synthesizing tissues in animals (23). It is also an active site of
carbohydrate metabolism (24,25,26,27). Since studies in our
laboratory and in others have shown that skin contains an active
prostaglandin synthetase activity for the conversion of arachidonic
acid into PGE_2 (28,29,30,31), we have examined the effects of
PGE_1, PGE_2, and insulin on carbohydrate metabolism in this tissue.

The effects of these three substances, added in vitro, on the
oxidation of uniformly ^{14}C-labelled glucose into CO_2 are shown in
Figure 1. Insulin (0.5 U/ml) and PGE_2 (0.5 µg/ml) significantly

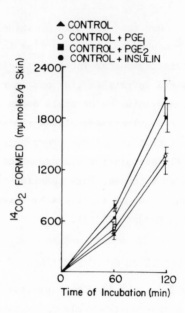

FIG. 1.   Effects of insulin, PGE_1, and PGE_2 on the oxidation of $[U-^{14}C]$glucose by rat skin.   Rat skin (50-100 mg) was incubated at 37° in 2.0 ml of Krebs-Ringer bicarbonate solution (pH 7.4) which contained 5 mM glucose, gentamicin sulfate (200 μg) and was gassed with 95% O_2 and 5% CO_2.   Incubations were carried out with $[U-^{14}]$glucose (2.5μCi per flask) in the presence of PGE_2 (0.5μg/ml) and insulin (0.5 unit/ml). $[^{14}C]CO_2$ was collected as previously described (31).   The number of nmoles of $[^{14}C]CO_2$ was calculated by dividing the amount of $[^{14}C]$ in the $[^{14}C]CO_2$ by the specific activity of $[U-^{14}C]$glucose in the medium and multiplying by 6.   The data from the average of three experiments and the vertical bars indicate range.

enhanced the oxidation of glucose into CO_2, while PGE_1 (0.5 μg/ml) was least active.

In further experiments, the effects of insulin and PGE_2 on the incorporation of $[1-^{14}C]$ glucose and $[6-^{14}C]$ glucose into lipids were examined.   The results are shown in Figure 2.   After 2 hours of incubation, insulin and PGE_2 enhanced the incorporation of glucose carbon into lipid fractions.   Addition of insulin and PGE_2 simultaneously to the incubation mixture had no additive effect.

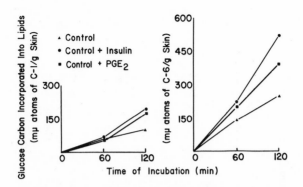

FIG. 2. Effects of insulin and PGE$_2$ on the incorporation of ^{14}C from [1-^{14}C]glucose and [6-^{14}C]glucose into lipids by rat skin. Methods of incubation are as described previously (28). The data were from the average of three experiments.

The effects of PGE$_2$ and insulin on the formation of fatty acids from [6-^{14}C]glucose and [1-^{14}C]glucose by rat skin in vitro were also examined. The data summarized in Table I indicate that PGE$_2$, like insulin, stimulated the flow of carbon from glucose into fatty acids. Addition of PGE$_2$ and insulin simultaneously to the incubation mixture did not cause any additive effect on the synthesis of fatty acids. Although PGE$_2$, like insulin, stimulated lipogenesis from glucose in rat skin, the precise mechanisms of action of PGE$_2$ in stimulating fatty acid synthesis in skin is not known and further studies are necessary to elucidate this point.

POSSIBLE ROLE IN SKIN OF EFA-DEFICIENT RATS

The nutritional requirement of mammalian species for certain fatty acids was first recognized in young rats and described by Burr and Burr (33,34). These investigators demonstrated that rats maintained on a fat-free diet over a long period developed an abnormality characterized by scaliness of the dorsal skin, feet, and tail, which subsequently became necrotic. These investigators proposed that linoleic and possibly linolenic were essential fatty acids (EFA).

TABLE I

Effects of Insulin and PGE$_2$ on Fatty Acid Synthesis from Glucose by Rat Skin In Vitro[a]

Addition	Glucose Carbon incorporated, mμatoms/hr/g Skin		
	All carbon	Carbon-1	Carbon-6
None	66 ± 3.8	18 ± 4.1	27 ± 5.2
Insulin (0.5 U/ml)	102 ± 17.4	36 ± 8.2	46 ± 10.4
PGE$_2$ (0.5 μg/ml)	91 ± 10.2	22 ± 6.7	37 ± 9.3
Insulin (0.5 U/ml) + PGE$_2$ (0.5 μg/ml)	108 ± 20.2	36 ± 8.8	49 ± 11.2

[a]Skin specimens from the same rats were incubated for 2 hours with glucose-U-^{14}C, glucose-1-^{14}C or glucose-6-^{14}C in 2 ml of Krebs-Ringer bicarbonate buffer (pH 7.4), containing 5 mM glucose and the antibiotic gentamicin sulfate. The number of mμ atoms of glucose carbon was calculated from the specific activity of the differentially labelled glucose in the medium, and the amount of ^{14}C incorporated into the acidic fraction obtained after hydrolysis of the neutral lipid fraction. (Each value represents the mean ± SD of the determinations from three rats.)

Although arachidonic acid is not a normal component in vege-
able fats, it is considered to be the principal unsaturated fatty
acid required by the animal organism.   Since studies have demonstrated that the essential fatty acids can be transformed enzymati-
cally into prostaglandins by homogenates and particulate fractions
of several tissues (35,36,37), including skin (28,29,30), we investigated whether prostaglandins do play any role in the syndrome of
EFA deficiency.

EFA deficiency was induced in male weanling rats according to
the procedure of Aaes-Jørgensen and Holman (38).   The experimental

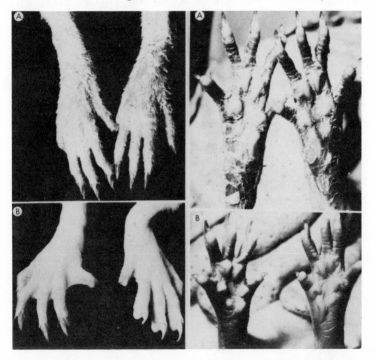

FIG. 3.   Effect of PGE₂ on scaly lesions of EFA-deficient rats.
A, severe scaling on the dorsum of the hind limbs of an EFA-deficient rat remains after two weeks of daily topical treatment with
propylene glycol:ethanol, 3:7 (v/v); B, clearance of the lesions
after two weeks of daily topical treatment with PGE₂ (100 µg) dissolved in propylene glycol:ethanol, 3:7 (v/v); C, severe scaling on
the plantar surface of the hind limbs of an EFA-deficient rat remains after two weeks of daily topical treatment with PGE₂ (100 µg)
dissolved in propylene glycol:ethanol, 3:7 (v/v).

group of animals were fed, ad lib, the basal diet supplemented with
hydrogenated coconut oil; the diet of the control animals was supplemented with safflower oil. The animals were housed in individual cages and maintained as described previously (32).

In all animals fed the basal diet supplemented with hydrogenated coconut oil, signs of EFA deficiency appeared after 6 to 8
weeks, with increasing severity in scaliness in the skin as the
experiment continued.

EFFECTS OF PGE$_2$ ON SKIN OF NORMAL AND EFA-DEFICIENT RATS

Intraperitoneal administration of 1 mg PGE$_2$ dissolved in 0.1
ml of saline/kg body weight did not clear the scaly lesions. This
lack of effect was probably due to rapid systemic metabolism of
PGE$_2$ to biologically inactive metabolites (39). Topical treatment
of the lesions with PGE$_2$ (100 µg/day) dissolved in a 3 to 7 (v/v)
propylene glycol-ethanol mixture cleared the scaly lesions in
approximately 14 days (Fig. 3). In another experiment, each EFA-
deficient rat was treated on one limb with PGE$_2$ dissolved in vehicle, and with vehicle alone on the other limb. The results
showed that the scaly lesions cleared in the PGE$_2$ treated limb and
not on the vehicle treated limb (Fig. 4). These results demonstrate that the action of PGE$_2$ in vivo is a local one and is not
transmitted via systemic circulation.

EFFECTS OF PGE$_2$ ON LIPID SYNTHESIS IN NORMAL AND EFA-DEFICIENT RATS

Incubation of skin specimens from normal and EFA-deficient
rats with [U-^{14}C]glucose showed an increase of ^{14}C incorporation from glucose into neutral lipids in skin of EFA-deficient
rats (Fig. 5). Fractionation of the neutral lipids into seven
fractions of Florisil columns (40) showed a 4- to 5-fold increase
of ^{14}C incorporated into sterol and wax ester fraction of EFA-
deficient rats (Fig. 6).

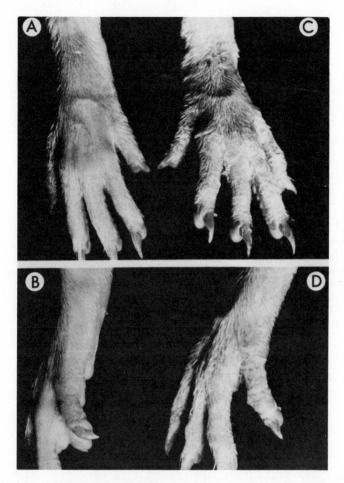

FIG. 4. Application of PGE$_2$ and vehicle to scaly hind limbs of the same rat. A and B, clearance of scaly lesions on the dorsum of one hind leg of an EFA-deficient rat after two weeks of daily topical treatment with PGE$_2$ (100 µg) dissolved in the vehicle; C and D, change in scaly lesions on the dorsum of the other hind leg of an EFA-deficient rat after two weeks of daily topical treatment with the vehicle.

The suggestion that increased esterification might be related to abnormal keratinization in the skin (41,42) spurred us to examine the effects of PGE$_2$ in vitro on the incorporation of ^{14}C from glucose into sterol esters. When skin from EFA-deficient and normal rats were incubated in the presence of $[$U-^{14}C$]$glucose and PGE$_2$, the incorporation of ^{14}C from labelled glucose into the sterol ester fraction of EFA-deficient rats was markedly

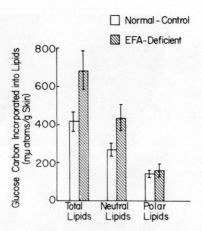

FIG. 5. Incorporation of glucose-U-^{14}C into lipids by skin of normal and EFA-deficient rats. Methods of incubation and recovery of lipids are as described under Fig. 1. The number of nano atoms of glucose carbon was calculated by dividing the amount of ^{14}C in the lipids by the specific activity of glucose-U-^{14}C in the medium and multiplying by 6. The data were the average of three experiments ± S.D.

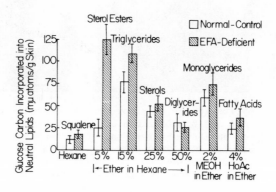

FIG. 6. Incorporation of glucose-U-^{14}C into neutral lipids by skin or normal and EFA-deficient rats. The neutral lipids were separated from Florisil columns, as described previously (32). The data were from the average of three experiments ± S.D. The abbreviations are: SQ, squalene; STEST, sterol and wax esters; TG, triglycerides; ST, sterols; DG, diglycerides; MG, monoglycerides; and FA, fatty acids.

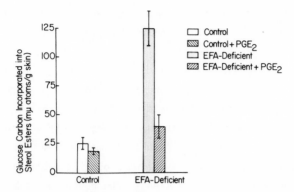

FIG. 7.   Inhibition of sterol ester synthesis of PGE_2. PGE_2
(0.5 µg/ml) was added to the incubation mixture consisting of
Krebs-Ringer bicarbonate buffer (pH 7.4), antibiotic, skin from
normal or EFA-deficient rats and glucose-U-^{14}C (5µCi, 0.36 µmole).
The amounts of ^{14}C incorporated from radioactive glucose into
neutral lipid fractions were determined by the procedures described
previously (32).   The data were obtained from the average of three
experiments ± S.D.

suppressed (Fig. 7).   This result is in harmony with reports des-

cribing the inhibitory effects of PGE_1 on cholesterol esterifi-

cation in the liver (43) and of $PGE_{2\alpha}$ in the corpus luteum (44).

A slight, but not too significant decrease was observed with skin

from normal control rats.   This difference between both specimens

could be due to the increased transcutaneous permeability in the

EFA-deficient rats, thus permitting easier penetration of PGE_2.

Whether the clearance of the scaly lesions in the skin of the

EFA-deficient rats is directly related to the inhibitory action of

PGE_2 on the biosynthesis of sterol esters cannot be determined by

the present data; nevertheless, the results do imply, however, that

PGE_2 plays a role in normalizing the scaly lesions induced by

EFA deficiency.   These results suggest possible connections between

arachidonic acid, PGE_2 and keratinization.

In conclusion, the regulation of the turnover of sterol esters

in the skin by PGE_2 is of particular interest.   In man, the re-

lationship of sterol esterification to keratinization has been

suggested by reports of reduced ratios of esterified sterols to

free sterols in psoriatic lesions (45), and in scales (46). Perhaps, one of the metabolic roles of PGE_2 in the skin, at least in
part, could be the maintenance of a balance between free and esterified sterols; such an assumption must, however, be verified.
The direct effects of prostaglandins on the enzyme systems involved
with the synthesis and hydrolysis of sterol esters are now under
study with the hope of elucidating the regulatory role of prostaglandins on enzymes involved with lipid metabolism. Our ultimate
hope of full understanding of the physiological role of these
potent endogenous substances lies in the continued efforts to
elucidate their mechanisms of action on metabolic processes.

ACKNOWLEDGMENTS

The author is grateful to Dr. John E. Pike of Upjohn Co. for
the generous supply of prostaglandins. The excellent technical
assistance of Mrs. Carmen Marquez and Mr. Rudy Guerra is gratefully
appreciated.

This investigation was supported in part by Grant AM 14941
of the U.S. Public Health Service and a research grant from
Hoffman-La Roche, Nutley, New Jersey.

REFERENCES

1. S. Bergstrom, L. A. Carlson, J. R. Weeks, Pharmacol. Rev., 20:
   1 (1968).

2. P. W. Ramwell and J. E. Shaw, in "Recent progress in hormone
   research," vol. 26, ed. E. B. Astwood, Academic Press, New
   York, 1970, p. 139.

3. D. Steinberg, M. Vaughan, P. J. Nestel, O. Strand, and
   S. Bergstrom, J. Clin. Invest., 43: 1533 (1964).

4. D. Steinberg, M. Vaughan, P. J. Nestel, Biochem. Pharmacol.,
   12: 764 (1963).

5. S. Bergstrom and L. A. Carlson, Acta Physiol. Scand., 63: 195
   (1963).

6. D. Steinberg and M. Vaughan, in "Novel symposium 2: prostaglandins," eds. S. Bergstrom and B. Samuelsson, Almquist and
   Wiksell, Stockholm; Interscience, New York, 1967, p. 109.

7. M. Vaughan and D. Steinberg, "Handbook of Physiology," eds.
    E. A. Renold and G. F. Cahill, Jr., American Physiological
    Society, Washington, D.C., 1965, p. 239.

8. M. Vaughan, J. E. Berger, and D. Steinberg, J. Biol. Chem.,
    239: 401 (1964).

9. O. Strand, M. Vaughan, and D. Steinberg, J. Lipid Res., 5: 554
    (1964).

10. F. P. Kupiecki, J. Lipid Res., 7: 230 (1966).

11. W. N. Spellacy, W. C. Buhi, and K. K. Holsinger, Amer. J.
    Obstet. Gynecol., 111: 239 (1971).

12. F. Bearti, N. Kabir, M. Naimzada, R, Lentati, P. Mantegazza,
    and R. Paoletti, Progr. Biochem. Pharmacol., 3: 110 (1967).

13. F. P. Kupiecki, J. Lipid Res., 8: 577 (1967).

14. E. Bohle, R. Dobert, and I. M. Merki, Z. Gesamte Exp. Med.,
    144: 285 (1967).

15. S. Bergstrom, L. A. Carlson, L. G. Ekelund, and L. Oro,
    Proc. Soc. Exp. Biol. Med., 118: 110 (1965).

16. S. Bergstrom, L. A. Carlson, and L. Oro, Acta Physiol. Scand.,
    67: 141 (1966).

17. L. A. Carlson, Progr. Biochem. Pharmacol., 3: 94 (1967).

18. E. Bohle and B. May, in "Prostaglandin symposium of the
    Worcester foundation for experimental biology," eds. P. W.
    Ramwell and J. E. Shaw, Interscience, New York, 1967, p. 115.

19. J. D. Crawford and H. A. Haessler, in "Prostaglandin sympo-
    sium of Worcester foundation for experimental biology," eds.
    P. W. Ramwell and J. E. Shaw, Interscience, New York, 1967,
    p. 103.

20. M. Vaughan, Prostaglandins, Proc. Novel Sym. 2nd, p. 139
    (1967).

21. C. H. Beatly and R. M. Bocek, Endocrinology, 90: 1295 (1971).

22. R. H. Swingert, C. E. Wagner, G. H. Herbener, and W. B.
    Atkinson, Endocrinology, 70: 600 (1962).

23. P. A. Srere, I. L. Chaikoff, S. S. Treitman, and L. S.
    Burnstein, J. Biol. Chem., 182: 629 (1950).

24. H. J. Yardley and G. Godfrey, Biochem. J., 86: 101 (1963).

25. K. M. Halprin and A. Ohkawara, J. Invest. Dermatol., 46: 43
    (1966).

26. S. H. Pomerantz and M. J. Asbornsen, Arch. Biochem. Biophys.,
    92: 147 (1961).

27. V. A. Ziboh, R. Wright, and S. L. Hsia, Arch. Biochem. Biophys.
    146: 93 (1971).

28. V. A. Ziboh and S. L. Hsia, Arch. Biochem. Biophys., 146: 100 (1971).

29. D. A. van Corp, Ann. N.Y. Acad. Sci., 180: 181 (1971).

30. C. E. Jonsson and E. Anggard, Scand. J. Clin. Lab. Invest., 29: 289 (1972).

31. V. A. Ziboh, J. Lipid Res., 14: 377 (1973).

32. V. A. Ziboh and S. L. Hsia, J. Lipid Res., 13: 458 (1972).

33. G. O. Burr and M. M. Burr, J. Biol. Chem., 82: 345 (1929).

34. G. O. Burr and M. M. Burr, J. Biol. Chem., 86: 587 (1930).

35. D. A. van Dorp, R. K. Beerthius, D. H. Nugteren, and H. von Keman, Biochim. Biophys. Acta, 90: 204 (1964).

36. S. Bergstrom, H. Danielsson, and B. Samuelsson, Biochim. Biophys. Acta, 90: 207 (1964).

37. E. J. Christ and D. H. Nugteren, Biochim. Biophys. Acta, 218: 296 (1970).

38. E. Aaes-Jorgensen and R. T. Holman, J. Nutr., 65: 633 (1958).

39. S. H. Ferreira and J. R. Vane, Nature (London), 216: 868 (1967).

40. K. K. Carroll, J. Lipid Res., 2: 135 (1961).

41. P. G. Unna and L. Golodetz, Biochem. Z., 25: 425 (1910).

42. D. J. Kooyman, Arch. Dermatol. 25: 444 (1932).

43. J. S. Schweppe and R. A. Jungmann, Proc. Soc. Exp. Biol. Med., 133: 1307 (1970).

44. H. R. Behrmann, G. J. MacDonald and R. O. Greep, Lipids, 6: 791 (1971).

45. A. Marchionini, E. Manz, and F. Huss, Arch. Dermatol. Syph., 176: 613 (1938).

46. R. P. Reinertston and V. R. Wheatley, J. Invest. Dermatol., 32: 49 (1959).

CHAPTER 20

PROSTAGLANDIN ANTAGONISTS

Kenneth E. Eakins

Department of Ophthalmology
Columbia University
New York, N.Y.

Over the years many specific antagonists of naturally occurring biologically active substances, such as acetylcholine, catecholamines, histamine, and 5-hydroxytryptamine have been developed, leading to many potent and clinically useful drugs. Recently, we have all been bombarded with a volumunous literature on the pharmacological effects and potential clinical usefulness of the prostaglandins and their analogs. However as evidence accumulates linking the endogenous prostaglandins to a variety of physiological and pathological conditions, we are beginning to realize the therapeutic potential of compounds that exhibit the actions and/or the synthesis of the prostaglandins.

The following is primarily concerned with the compounds that antagonize the action of the PG's, but I will also discuss inhibitors of synthesis. Several PG antagonists are available but the present-day compounds are not universally effective and only some of them have an adequate degree of selectivity. There are three main groups of compounds available at the present time, namely, the prostaglandin analogs such as 7-oxa-13-prostynoic acid, developed by Fried and coworkers in Chicago (1); SC 19220, a dibenzoxazepine derivative developed at G. D. Searle and Company and described by John Sanner (2); and polyphloretin phosphate and related compounds, stumbled across by Karim and myself (3).

Most studies with these antagonists have been based on the
ability to inhibit contractions of intestinal muscle induced by PGE
and PGF compounds but, as we will see, experiments in other tissues
have produced valuable results as well. The drug, 7-oxa-13-
prostynoic acid, was developed classically by modification of the
agonist or prostaglandin molecule. This drug antagonizes PGE and F
compounds in different tissues, but, according to Flack (4), it
appears to be selective only in the gerbil colon. It did not
antagonize contractions produced by prostaglandins on human isolated
gut muscle (5). SC 19220 is also a selective antagonist of PGE_2-
and $PGF_{2\alpha}$-induced contractions on animal gastrointestinal tissues,
but as with 7-oxa-13-prostynoic acid, SC 19220 is ineffective on
human isolated gut. The third antagonist, polyphloretin phosphate
(PPP), is a mixture of polyesters of phloretin and phosphoric acid.
This drug antagonizes contractions produced by PGE_2 and $PGF_{2\alpha}$ on
most tissues and it is the only one that Bennett and Posner (5)
found to be effective on human gut. In their study PPP was found
to be effective in every tissue except the rat fundus, where,
interestingly, it produces a dose-dependent contraction. In addition, PPP has been of use in the development of a specific assay
for angiotensin, using the isolated rat colon to block the effects
of PG's present in bioassay samples (6). One more interesting
point arises from these smooth-muscle studies: none of these
antagonists would inhibit a relaxation produced by a prostaglandin
(for example, that produced by PGE_2 in circular muscle strips),
indicating that there are at least two types of receptors for PGE
compounds, and that no antagonist is available for the type of
receptor mediating smooth-muscle relaxation. Similarly, no antagonist has been found to block the PGE-induced relaxation of
isolated human bronchi.

Mathe et al. (7) demonstrated that PPP could selectively
block contractions produced by $PGF_{2\alpha}$ on an isolated human bronchial
strip. Clinically, this is of potential interest in view of the
possible involvement of endogenous $PGF_{2\alpha}$ in anaphyllaxis, with its

attendant bronchoconstriction.   In a further study on the isolated
human bronchi preparation, Mathe and Strandberg (8) showed that PPP
could also antagonize the bronchoconstrictor effects of purified
slow-reacting substance (SRS) without modifying the bronchoconstriction produced by either acetylcholine or histamine.   Both SC 19220
and PPP have been found to prevent the diarrhoea induced by intraperitoneal injections of PGE_2 in mice (9,10).   It has been suggested that PG's are involved in the pathogenesis of different
forms of diarrhoea; thus, antagonists may be of potential value in
the treatment of this condition.

Figure 1 is taken from a study on the anesthetized cat to
illustrate some of the complexities of PG antagonism (11).   We see
that $PGF_{2\alpha}$ increases intraileal pressure, increases airway pressure

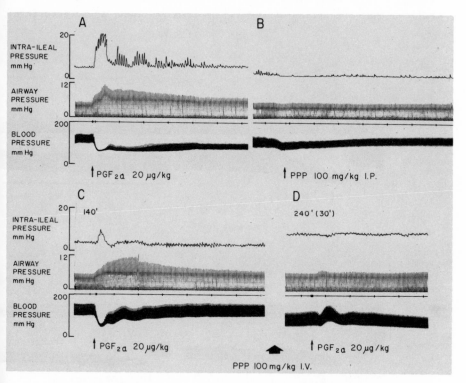

FIG. 1.   Separation of inhibitory effects of PPP on responses
to $PGF_{2\alpha}$.   A, control responses to $PGF_{2\alpha}$ (20µg/kg i.v.); B, responses to PPP (100 mg/kg i.p.); C, responses to $PGF_{2\alpha}$ (20µg/kg i.v.)
140 minutes after i.p. PPP; D, responses to $PGF_{2\alpha}$ (20µg/kg i.v.) 30
minutes after a second dose of PPP (100 mg/kg i.v.).   (From Ref. 11.)

and decreases blood pressure. Following the intraperitoneal injection of 100 mg/kg PPP, the gut response is markedly decreased,
as is the fall in blood pressure, but the airway pressure response
is intact. However, following an intravenous injection of a
further 100 mg/kg PPP, all three responses are virtually abolished.
In contrast (Fig. 2), we see that with PGE_2 the gut's response is
abolished following intravenous injection of a large dose of PPP,
but the fall in blood pressure is not. If anything, the fall in
blood pressure is more prolonged. Similar results were obtained in
the anesthetized dog by White and Pennink (12). In this species,
$PGF_{2\alpha}$ caused a pressor response; following PPP this was reversed to
a prolonged depressor response. However, the depressor response to
PGE_2 was clearly enhanced by the PPP. These results lead us to
believe that the action of PPP is complex, and that it can interfere

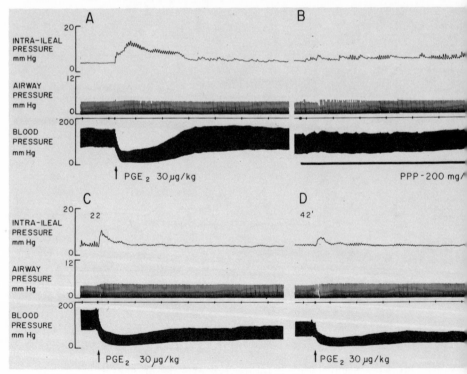

FIG. 2. Inhibition by PPP of ileal response to PGE_2. A,
control responses to PGE_2 (30µg/kg i.v.); B, response to PPP (200
mg/kg i.v.); C and D, inhibition of ileal response to PGE_2 22 and
42 minutes after PPP. (From Ref. 11.)

with the metabolism of the prostaglandins. Certainly, Marrazzi and
Matschinsky (13) have shown that PPP is a competitive inhibitor of
the PG binding site with respect to prostaglandin 15-dehydrogenase,
an enzyme of crucial importance in the degradation of prostaglandins. Interestingly, 7-oxa-13-prostynoic acid also inhibited in
this system, but SC 19220 did not. It is therefore apparent that
results with PPP or other antagonists may be complicated by this
effect, and the potency as a blocker may be decreased if the target
organ or tissue has a lot of PG dehydrogenase activity.

Some antagonists have been shown to inhibit the effects of
PG's on the adenyl-cyclase/cyclic-AMP system in various tissues and
to modify the effect of the hormone stimulus (Table I). In this
way they have been used to study the participation of PG's as
intermediaries in the process of hormonal action. Note that one
either blocks or enhances hormonal action depending on whether or
not the PG's increase or decrease the cyclic-AMP levels in the
tissue.

I would now like to deal briefly with the possible clinical
use of prostaglandin antagonists as anti-inflammatory agents.

TABLE I

Some Tissues in which PG Antagonists Block the Effects of PG's
on the Cyclic AMP System and Modify Hormonal Action

Tissue	Effect of PG on cyclic AMP	Hormone	PG antagonist	Effect of hormonal response	Ref. No.
Ovary (mouse)	+	LH	7-oxa-13-prostynoic acid	Block	(14)
Ovary (rat)	+	LH	PPP	Block	(15)
Bladder (toad)	−	ADH	7-oxa-13-prostynoic acid PPP (SC 19220 - no effect)	Enhance	(16)
Thyroid (bovine)	+	TSH	7-oxa-13-prostynoic acid PPP	Block	(17) (18)

There is now increasing evidence that PG's may be important in the
inflammatory response (19). The eye is one organ in which we feel
that PG's play a significant role in the mediation of the acute
inflammatory response (20). Exogenous PG's can produce many of
the signs of ocular inflammation both in experimental animals and
man, including vasodilation, increased vascular permeability
(manifested as an increase in the protein content of the aqueous
humour), and a raised intraocular pressure. We studied the effect
of topical PG's on the anterior uvea in the absence and presence of
PPP using fluorescein iris angiography, a very sensitive indicator
of vascular permeability (21). In Figure 3 we can see the same eye

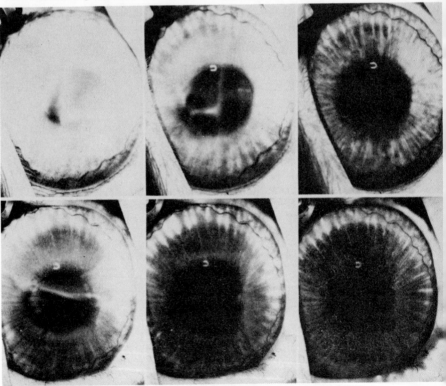

FIG. 3.   Antagonism by polyphloretin phosphate of the increase
in permeability produced by prostaglandin E_1 (0.025%). Eye treated
topically with prostaglandin E_1 alone (left) and then with prostaglandin E_1 in the presence of polyphloretin phosphate (right).
Angiographic appearances at one minute (top), five minutes (center),
and ten minutes (bottom). (From Ref. 21.)

of the same rabbit, treated on different occasions with topical
PGE_1 alone and with both PGE_1 and a subconjunctival injection of
10 mg PPP. Fluorescein was injected intravenously and photographs
taken at set intervals using a motorized Nikon F 35 mm camera.
Comparing the PPP-treated eye with the control, we can see that at
1 minute, there is less fluorescence of the radial iris vessels;
at 5 minutes, the same difference holds true and there is no
fluorescein in the anterior chamber; at 10 minutes, there is
markedly less fluorescein in the anterior chamber of the PPP-
treated eye, indicating a substantial decrease in the permeability
of the blood vessels produced by the prostaglandin.

It is obvious from my remarks that these first-generation
prostaglandin antagonists must be considered as starting points for
the development of more potent and selective compounds. In fact,
there is a great effort being made along these lines. However,
these present compounds have been of use as pharmacological tools
in studies concerned with the physiological roles of prostaglandins, and they have indicated several areas of possible clinical
application for the group as a whole—such as the control of gastrointestinal motility and diarrhoea, management of certain forms of
bronchoconstriction, and as anti-inflammatory agents (particularly
in the skin and eye). Furthermore, we have learned that it is not
possible to extrapolate data from one species, or even one tissue,
to another. Hence, I do not feel that we will see the development
of an overall blocker of the actions of PG's at every site in the
body. Rather, we will end up with agents which are very tissue
and specie specific.

The second group of drugs that must be considered are those
which inhibit the synthesis of prostaglandins. Nonsteroidal anti-
inflammatory agents such as aspirin and indomethacin were found to
inhibit the biosynthesis of prostaglandins (22,23,24). It has been
suggested that this inhibition of prostaglandin biosynthesis by
aspirin is the mechanism by which aspirin exerts its anti-inflammatory, analgesic, and and antipyretic actions. Steroidal

anti-inflammatory agents such as dexamethasone, hydrocortisone,
and fludrocortisone may also interfere somewhere in the PG system,
but not by direct synthetase inhibition (even at concentrations of
100 µg/ml these steroids gave less than a 10% inhibition of PG
biosynthesis in the microsomal preparations of dog spleen (25).
Furthermore, aldosterone, a steroid which is not anti-inflammatory,
had the same weak activity against PG biosynthesis as dexamethasone.
A variety of other compounds were also tested and found to be
inactive, indicating that inhibition of PG biosynthesis is therefore a unique characteristic of aspirinlike anti-inflammatory drugs.
Aspirin and indomethacin have been used extensively as pharmacological tools to study the role of PG's in many physiological and
pathological conditions. For example, work with these compounds
has added much evidence on the role of prostaglandins in the production of inflammation, pain, and fever, and in adrenergic neuro-
transmission, maintenance of smooth-muscle tone, kidney function,
and reproduction.

However, as with the receptor antagonists, selectivity is not
yet absolute. Many people are using these agents as pharmacological tools without even considering the possibility that compounds,
such as aspirin and indomethacin, may have actions other than on
PG biosynthesis, and this may not be wise. For example, Flores and
Sharp (26) have recently shown in the toad bladder that indomethacin can exhibit phosphodiesterase. In fact, on these toad-bladder
homogenates indomethacin was more potent than theophylline in this
respect. More caution should be exercised in interpreting the
physiological roles of PG's from experiments with these inhibitors.

As with the PG antagonists, the next generation of synthetase
inhibitors will be more specie and organ specific. Experimental
evidence for this comes from studies by Flower and Vane (27) on the
anomalous behaviour of the antipyretic, paracetamol. This is a
compound which has no anti-inflammatory activity, but is analgesic
and antipyretic. It had little effect on PG synthetase derived
from dog spleen, whereas it was active against rabbit-brain

synthetase.   In contrast, indomethacin was much less active as an
inhibitor of PG biosynthesis in brain tissue than in spleen.   The
authors concluded that their results illustrated the mechanism by
which the clinical actions of the aspirinlike drugs are determined
by the differential sensitivity of the PG-synthetase systems of
the target organ.   This sort of result is important.   For example,
PG's can decrease gastric secretion and have even been proposed for
use in the treatment of gastric ulcers; thus, we do not want to
inhibit formation of PG's in the gastrointestinal tract.   The differential data shows us that we can look for an inhibitor for use
as an antipyretic or anti-inflammatory agent which will not produce
the gastrointestinal side effects which are a major drawback to the
use of aspirin.

Study of the PG-synthetase systems from different tissues will
lead to aspirinlike drugs with a much greater specificity of action,
and study of inhibitors which act at different sites in the
PG-biosynthetic pathway may yield inhibitors which block the
formation of either E or F PG's rather than both together.

In conclusion, I would like to reiterate that the inability
of an antagonist to block the effects of PG's everywhere, or the
inability of a synthetase inhibitor to block all synthetase
systems to the same extent, is not a drawback.   Indeed, the reverse
is true, since it opens up the possibility of developing compounds
with a high degree of tissue specificity.

REFERENCES

1.   J. Fried, T. S. Santhanakrishnan, J. Himizu, C. H. Lin,
     S. H. Ford, S. Rubin, and E. O. Grigas, Nature (London), 223:
     208 (1969).

2.   J. H. Sanner, Arch. Int. Pharmacodyn. Ther., 180: 46 (1969).

3.   K. E. Eakins, S. M. M. Karim, and J. D. Miller, Brit. J.
     Pharmacol., 39: 556 (1970).

4.   J. D. Flack, Recent Prog. Horm. Res., 26: 174 (1970).

5.   A. Bennett and J. Posner, Brit. J. Pharmacol., 42: 584 (1971).

6. D. J. Gagnon and P. Sirois, Brit. J. Pharmacol., 46: 89 (1972).

7. A. A. Mathe, K. Strandberg, and A. Astrom, Nature New Biol., 230: 215 (1971).

8. A. A. Mathe and K. Strandberg, Acta Physiol. Scand., 82: 460 (1971).

9. J. H. Sanner, Intra-sci. Chem. Rep., 6: 1 (1972).

10. K. E. Eakins, Ann. N.Y. Acad. Sci., 180: 386 (1971).

11. R. Villaneuva, L. Hinds, R. L. Katz and K. E. Dakins, J. Pharmacol., 180: 78 (1972).

12. R. P. White and M. Pennink, Arch. Int. Pharmacodyn. Ther., 197: 274 (1972).

13. M. A. Marrazzi and F. M. Matschinsky, Prostaglandins, 1: 373 (1972).

14. F. A. Kuehl, J. L. Humes, J. Tarnoff, V. J. Cirillo, and E. A. Ham, Science, 169: 883 (1970).

15. T. Perklev and K. Ahren, Life Sci., 10: 1387 (1971).

16. A. Ozer and G. W. G. Sharp, Amer. J. Physiol., 222: 674 (1972).

17. G. Burke, K. Kowalski, and D. Babiarz, Life Sci., 10: 513 (1971).

18. S. Sato, K. Kowalski, and G. Burke, Prostaglandins, 1: 345 (1972).

19. A. L. Willis, P. Davison, P. W. Ramwell, W. E. Brocklehurt, and B. Smith, in "Prostaglandins in cellular biology," eds. P. W. Ramwell and B. B. Pharriss, Plenum Press, New York, 1972, pp. 227-259.

20. K. E. Eakins in "The prostaglandins," Vol. 1, ed. P. W. Ramwell, Plenum Press, New York, 1973, pp. 219-237.

21. R. A. F. Whitelocke and K. E. Eakins, Arch. Ophthalmol., 89: 495 (1973).

22. J. R. Vane, Nature New Biol., 231: 232 (1971).

23. J. B. Smith and A. L. Willis, Nature New Biol., 231: 235 (1971).

24. S. H. Ferreira, S. Moncada, and J. R. Vane, Nature New Biol., 231: 237 (1971).

25. R. Flower, R. Gryglewski, K. Herbaczynska-Cedro, and J. R. Vane, Nature New Biol., 238: 104 (1972).

26. A. G. A. Flores and G. W. G. Sharp, Amer. J. Physiol., 233: 1392 (1972).

27. R. Flower and J. R. Vane, Nature, 240: 410 (1972).

CHAPTER 21

PROTOCOL DESIGN
A PANEL DISCUSSION

Discussion Participants

Roger F. Palmer, Professor and Chairman, Department of Pharmacology, University of Miami School of Medicine, Miami, Florida.

C. Paul Bianchi, Professor, Department of Pharmacology, University of Pennsylvania School of Medicine, Philadelphia, Pennsylvania.

Dean J. Clyde, President, Clyde Computing Service, Miami, Florida.

Stephen L. DeFelice, President, Clinical Resources, Inc., New York, New York.

Harvey L. Dickstein, Associate Director, Department of Clinical Research, Abbot Laboratories, North Chicago, Illinois.

James A. Hagans, Chief of Cooperative Studies Program, Veterans Administration Hospital, Miami, Florida.

Roger G. Mazlen, Assistant Director of Clinical Research, Ayerst Laboratories, New York, New York.

F. Gilbert McMahon, Professor and Chairman, Therapeutics Section, Tulane University School of Medicine, New Orleans, Louisiana.

Milton M. Willner, Director of Medical Research, Hoffman-La Roche Inc., Nutley, New Jersey.

231

DR. PALMER: This morning we have a panel discussion on how to
design a protocol, which is a title that is way too ambitious. We
talked about it briefly in terms of how some units go about designing a protocol. Dr. McMahon's slide with the big cloud of the FDA
sitting over it, I hope, isn't sitting over us today when we begin
discussing the scientific basis of protocol design. We can confine
ourselves to Phase I, Phase II, or Phase III, but since this is a
discussion of the first human dose, maybe we can concentrate on
Phase I.

I have my own ideas of how to proceed in getting together the
kinds of minds to look at the problem, which I mentioned in the
first part of the symposium. There are others. Dr. DeFelice will
talk about how he thinks people ought to get together to design a
protocol. The questions that one begins to consider at this stage
are: What type of patients? Should we use normal volunteers?
How many patients should one study? Should there be a few well-
studied patients, or should one take a large number? Is pharmacokinetic data necessary? Should we have it in the prehuman work?
We've heard views from Ken Melmon and others that perhaps it is
desirable to have it not only in the Phase I study, but also to
have animal pharmacokinetic data prior to the first human dose.
How do you go about picking the first human dose? Should there be
an anaphylactic test dose? We in our clinic uniformly give an absurdly low dose just to make sure there isn't some more anaphylactic peculiarity in the human. Does one push to the therapeutic
effect, or should one go beyond it and get the desired toxic effect
in Phase I? Is it necessary to expose a human being to the toxic
effect if there are good animal data to tell you what the toxic
effect will be? What is the introduction of bias by patient
selection? Is there an inherent bias in asking somebody to

volunteer? There are studies indicating that the volunteer has a
different psychological profile than the rest of his colleagues.
Is this valid data or not? Does the fact that prisoners get benefits and a few dollars mean that they will deny symptomatology?
These are some of the very broad problems that one must consider in
designing a protocol.

Then we have the problem of statistical design. Dr. Cohen has
asked Dr. Dean J. Clyde, author of the Clyde Mood Scale, to speak
to us. Dr. Clyde is presently head of the Clyde Computing Service
and was director of the biometric laboratory of George Washington
University from 1960 to 1963. He is now in Miami, and we're
fortunate to have him down here.

DR. CLYDE: There are two handouts on the back table. Don't
be turned off by the title. It's "Understanding Statistical
Analysis in Psychiatry," and it was given that title because it was
published in a psychiatric journal; but it could equally well be
titled, "Understanding Statistical Analysis in Medicine" or ".....
in Pharmacology." As a matter of fact, none of the statistical
methods discussed in the reprint were originally invented for
psychiatry or medicine. Most of them were developed in the field
of agriculture. R. A. Fisher was one of the world's leading
statisticians, who invented analysis of variance—and he invented
it for agriculture. We're now evaluating drugs in humans by the
same statistical methods that were used to evaluate fertilizers on
land in England. We've come a long way.

Protocol design is influenced by the statistical tools that
are available. There may be two ways of doing an experiment. One
way might make a lot of medical sense and be an excellent way to
collect data, but a statistician might advise you that there's no
way that he can apply statistics to the data and perform tests of
significance. The statistician may say that if you change the
experiment somewhat, if you modify your protocol design (sometimes
it's a small change, sometimes a drastic change), then he will have
the statistical tools to apply to your data and he can do tests of

significance. Sometimes both of these experimental designs make
sense, and this generates a conflict. You see it in professional
meetings when there are two different ways of doing things. Sometimes the investigator objects to modifying the design so that
statistical tools can be applied. In the field of clinical research, the investigator may say the modifications are unrealistic,
that is, you're forcing conditions on him which are not really
appropriate. The statistician says, "If you don't do it that way,
we can't draw any valid conclusions from the study."

I think that the existence of certain statistical tools has
generated a lot of this controversy. Plainly, if a statistical
tool does not exist for a certain type of problem it puts pressure
on the investigator not to use that approach, but some other
approach for which there is a statistical tool. We all know the
position of the FDA. The FDA will put tremendous pressure on you
to select a design for which there is a statistical tool, because
the other type of experiment has fallen out of favor. This means
that the availability of statistical tools can influence the kind
of protocol design you adopt. But we all should realize that statistics is not a static field. Statistics, as a field, is advanc-
ing. A statistical tool which we may not have had last year, we
may possess this year. So a protocol design which may have been
unacceptable last year because we did not have a statistical tool
for it, suddenly becomes acceptable because we do have a statistical tool. It seems to me, in the current climate of opinion,
particularly with the FDA favoring statistical analysis, it
behooves the investigator to know something about what tools are
available. There's a big cultural lag in this, like in everything
else. New statistical tools are invented which make possible new,
and I think better, protocol designs, and yet it may be years
before their availability filters through to clinical pharmacologists.

I'm going to mention just two examples of statistical tools
which can influence protocol design for the better, I think. The

fact that we have these statistical tools makes it possible for you
to do better, more realistic research. There are others which are
mentioned in that reprint on the back table. In one typical protocol in clinical pharmacology, let's suppose that we have a drug
which is supposed to affect the blood level of a certain chemical
in human beings. Typically, we'll take a number of humans; we'll
measure their blood level before treatment; we'll put them on this
drug; and we'll measure the blood levels at a number of intervals
after treatment begins. Let's say, for example, that we measure
the blood level before treatment and then we measure the blood
level of the chemical every day for 14 days while the patient is
undergoing treatment with the drug. Of course, the crucial thing
which tells us whether the drug is having an effect is the comparison of the patient's blood levels after treatment with those before
treatment. The problem is, in many studies, that we do not have an
accurate measurement of that pretreatment level. The unreliability
of clinical laboratories is notorious. The fact is that we've
gotten one pretreatment blood level, which may be very inaccurate,
and yet that's our baseline for comparing, let's say, 14 post- or
during-treatment intervals. If our baseline is sloppy, we may
draw erroneous conclusions about whether this drug is making blood
level go up or down. Mike Free, a statistician with Smith, Kline &
French, who has run into this problem many times, has done some
theoretical/mathematical studies as well as some practical ones,
and he has come up strong for having more than one pretreatment
measurement. If your pretreatment measurement is unreliable, you
can improve on it. If it fluctuates from day to day, or hour to
hour, you can get a more accurate measure if you measure it more
than once. By measuring it twice, on two days before treatment,
you get a much more accurate baseline than you would have if you
measured it just once. This assumes that the clinical measure does
vary from day to day and is subject to errors of measurement. Of
course, if you're measuring a patient's height, there probably is
no need to measure it more than once before treatment. But

unfortunately, an awful lot of the variables we deal with are not
measured that well, and so it definitely gives you a better baseline if you measure it twice or more. In the example where you
measure pretreatment once and posttreatment 14 times, say once each
day, I wouldn't go so far as to say you would have to measure pretreatment 14 times. I think that's probably overdetermining it,
but at least twice is often recommended.

It's not enough if you just measure it twice; if it's going to
be subjected to statistical analysis, those two measurements must
actually be used in the statistics. There's no use measuring it
twice if the statistician uses only one measurement. Until a few
years ago there was no good way to use more than one pretreatment
measure. The technique of analysis of covariance, which is the
technical name for making use of pretreatment measures, for many
years was limited to one pretreatment measure. The mathematical
theory for handling more than one was understood, but in practice
it was so much work that people didn't do it. Now computer programs exist which will handle multiple-baseline measurements. The
availability of computer programs to handle multiple-pretreatment
measures makes possible, in my mind, an improvement in protocol
design.

I'll choose another example of how the availability of statistical tools can lead to better conclusions. This is in the area of
cooperative studies. A lot of you, I suppose, just do studies on
your own. You collect data, you do whatever analysis is indicated,
and you publish it or give it to a drug company or the FDA. More
and more, we are all getting into cooperative studies, where the
data collected from a number of investigators from a number of
different locations must somehow be pooled and valid conclusions
drawn. If you never get involved in cooperative studies and you
don't plan to, you don't have to listen to what I'm going to say.
But if you have been involved in cooperative studies where there's
pooling of data, or you think you might be, my next remarks will
be apropos. There's been a lot of controversy over the correct way

to handle the data. Many clinicians have objected, rightly I think,
to simply lumping data from many different institutions together
and ignoring the fact that the data came from different institutions. They say the patients may be more severely ill in one
institution compared with another. And I agree.

The theoretical technique for coping statistically with data
from a number of different investigators was invented about 40
years ago by R. A. Fisher. He called it "the factorial experiment,"
and the statistical procedure for analyzing "the analysis of
variance." The factorial experiment can take into account the fact
that the data came from different hospitals, let's say. The yellow
handout is an example of real data of the type which has been
analyzed by the analysis or variance, which came from, in this case,
five different hospitals. On the first page, you will notice a
comment which says that differences among five hospitals are removed and do not affect evaluation of treatments. This was a study
in which there were two treatments being compared—an active treatment and a nontreatment, or control, in five hospitals. It
happened that the accumulation of suitable patients was rather slow
in these hospitals. So in order to speed up the accumulation of
data, we got five hospitals to agree on a common protocol. We
obtained before-treatment and after-treatment data on two treatments in five hospitals. The analysis of variance procedure for
the experiment was known in theory, but in practice there was one
difficulty. If you have equal numbers in each hospital, equal
numbers of patients in each treatment in each hospital, then the
analysis of variance of the pre- and post-scores is rather simple.
But, of course, in practice we almost never have equal numbers. We
may start out with that intention, but due to practical difficulties in clinical research, we end up with somewhat unequal numbers.
Furthermore, it's quite likely that one hospital may get the type
of patient we're looking for at a faster rate than another. If
they can study more patients, why not let them? Well, the theory
of analysis of variance with unequal numbers was known for a long

time, but in practice the computations were so formidable that
nobody did them. So no statistician would have advised that you do
this sort of experiment unless you could get equal numbers in each
set. This was a severe constraint and led to quite a lot of controversy.

I sat in on some protocol design meetings where this very fact
led to argument. They said, "The hell with statistics, let's collect the data even though the numbers are going to be unequal, and
let's draw our conclusions." For seven years now there has been a
computer program which can do the analysis of variance with unequal
numbers, and I mentioned that the theory was known long before that.
There is a computer program available; it was used for this particular example in the handout. If you look at the second page,
there's a column headed "N". This is the number of patients which
were actually in each cell. You can see one of the cells has 2
patients, another 20, another 11, and so on. As I mentioned, some
of the hospitals could get patients at a faster rate than others.
It's possible to do the analysis. You evaluate the difference
between treatments removing any difference among hospitals. You
don't want differences among hospitals to confound your evaluation
of treatments. The analysis of variance separates these two. You
actually get two tests of significance, one for determining if the
hospitals differ, and the other, which you're really interested in,
for determining if Treatment 1 is better than Treatment 2. It
turned out in this worked example that Treatment 1 was better than
Treatment 2, and also that there were very significant differences
among hospitals.

I have tried to point out two examples in which the development of statistical tools and the feasibility of using the tools,
because the computer programs are generally available, can influence protocol design for the better. The first example I gave was
that it may be wise in certain cases to take more than one baseline
measure. These can be entered into the statistical analysis and
usually render a more valid and precise result. The other is that

in cooperative studies where there are a number of investigators
collecting data with the same protocol, we don't just crudely pool
the data as if they were identical. It's possible to evaluate the
treatments while removing the differences from one investigator to
another. These are just two examples of statistical tools which
are available. There are others which may make it possible for you
to design and carry out better experiments. I think with every
year that passes you have fewer restrictions put on you by statistics. You have fewer restraints, and you may be able to do the
kind of research which you think is medically sensible and which a
statistician will also say is sensible.

DR. PALMER: Dr. DeFelice is president of an organization,
Clinical Resources, Inc., which is approaching the problem of protocol design in a unique way, I think.   I'd be very interested to
hear how his organization operates.

DR. DeFELICE: During the past few days you've heard about a
broad spectrum of obstacles to clinical research. When Dean Clyde
says there wasn't a statistical method around to handle two base-
lines, and it takes years for this procedure to come into being,
just imagine our present problems and what must still come into
being.

Can anyone deny that we have created a monster, where obstacles to clinical research continue to grow? Let's say we want to
do a study with a new compound emanating from a major pharmaceutical company. What do you face? You have FDA guidelines which
may be incorrect and limit the imagination; you might not have a
statistical method; you always have a potential litigation problem;
you must have peer-group review; you have problems of theoretical
toxicity; maybe it's a mutagen—you have all sorts of problems.
Each one spells delay, delay. We're seeing that today. How do you
cut through this gordion knot? How does one move forward with
vigor, and yet credibility? There's only one method that I can
think of, and that's the peer-group approach. This is the method
we're utilizing in our organization.

The philosophy is a simple one. What has happened in the late
60s and 70s is what I call the "opening up" of the Food and Drug
Administration. This means the peer-group review, where academia
exerts a significant influence on regulatory drug decisions and
clinical drug development. The pharmaceutical industry also has
its peer groups. Both the FDA and the industry, understandably,
have vested interests. What is needed therefore is another peer-
group mechanism that interfaces between the FDA and industry consultants.

The only way to establish credibility is to be good. Here's
how we do it. Let's say the FDA or a pharmaceutical company comes
to us with a problem—be it a new drug or a marketing one. What we
do is assemble five to ten authorities pertinent to the problem.
At times there are only a few physicians on the peer group.

We always have a statistician in high visibility, because
we're in Pythagorean times and the P value has replaced God and
common sense. The P value of .05 or less has been etched in
regulatory stone. What we do is run what we call a peer-group
analysis, which takes about 90 days. We go to the client, be it
the government, foundations, or the industry and we say, "Look,
you can't interact with our peer group." The FDA and the industry
almost always participate with their peer-group members during
deliberation. Now perhaps Aristotle and St. Francis can stay
neutral in this type of environment but the majority of men and
women cannot. The FDA, utilizing outside consultants, almost
always found fixed combinations to be bad. Similarly, the industry
almost always found them to be good. Now, who's kidding who? It
does not require a great syllogistic effort to conclude that some
are good and some are bad. This "clear thinking" can only be done
when decision making is sufficiently removed from the arena of
vested interest. In addition, our peer-group members are not permitted to perform studies emanating from the analysis. By isolating
the peer group and by excluding future studies we believe we have
fulfilled certain conditions of objectivity.

I am a firm believer in a Ph.D. approach in clinical research.
I think the M.D., if he's a good one, is worth his weight in gold.
You need that M.D. input. We have a M.D. to Ph.D. ratio of maybe
one to three and are shooting for one to four. The Ph.D. is
important because clinical research is more scientific and more
disciplined; this is what the Ph.D. is all about. Again, you need
that M.D. input. We usually assign one or two Ph.D.'s and one M.D.
to the peer-group team. We visit with the client, and discuss and
gather appropriate information. We put the peer-group package
together and submit it to the peer group. We're a "package-putter-
together", so to speak.

Then we run a 90-day program during which the peer-group members are worked very, very hard. We assemble them at our head-
quarters and they don't leave until the questions are answered. We
assemble them periodically—it can be two, three, or four times.
No one comes in and states that combinations are irrational. We
don't tolerate that kind of thinking. We say: Given the fact that
this is a combination, how do we test its rationality? We try to
eliminate unhealthy bias right from the beginning. Within a 90-day
period of time, the client receives a report, be it an NDA approach
or a product defense. Included are the rationale, protocols,
statistical approach, comments on probability, etc. We assess all
these factors in the final report. We have cut through the jungle
of problems effectively.

If it calls for international studies, we go. And we do it
well. The inference the other day was that if you go international,
you're immoral. This is an arrogant position. Anyway, we go
abroad, because answers supersede ideology. Do you have a product?
Is it a good product? Whatever questions one is asking about the
product, we'll try to answer them within a period of time such that
you don't have this absurd lag which is destroying inspiration and
thereby innovation. This is how we operate. And I'm predicting
that there will be many such private organizations by the mid-70s—
not to replace our present system, but as a means of goosing it, so
to speak.

DR. PALMER: We've had some provocative remarks. I'd like now
to call the panel to come forward. Gil McMahon, I wonder if you'd
be willing to come on up and sit up here, too.

DR. WILLNER: I'd like to direct my question primarily to
Dr. DeFelice. Let me start out by saying that we do not have any
prejudice against the use of private research organizations. We do
use them. But Dr. DeFelice's main pitch is that credibility is
somehow better if you use an organization of his type. I'm at a
loss to understand how that follows because, as the old adage says,
"He who pays the piper will call the tune." He's being paid by
somebody, not generating funds from the NIH or any so-called
impartial organization. I'd like him to tell me how his credibility
is better than anybody else's as long as there is a question of
bias because of the source of financial support.

DR. DeFELICE: That's something history will show us. Logical-
ly, you're right. We can be judged as a surrogate for a vested
interest, since there is no institution without such interests.
What I'm saying is that in our present environment we do have an
adversary group utilizing peer groups as position supporters. It
is leading to decisions which are not really healthy. There is no
mechanism in the culture to handle the problem of combination antibiotics dispassionately. The industry can't and the government
can't. What is the alternative? I'm saying one has to attempt our
approach in this culture at this point in time. And the proof of
the pudding is in what we do. Two or three years from now you'll
know.

DR. PALMER: Steve, let me say something about that, too. The
peer-review system at the NIH has been doing things for years,
trusting the integrity of the individual site visitor, if you will.
There are situations where (and we have a site visit coming up) the
site visitors who are evaluating your program are in competition
with you during the same fiscal years. Dr. Reuter, from Germany,
pointed out to me that this is probably a bad system. He would

suggest that we have foreigners come over to evaluate, since they
have no vested interest. On the other hand, I think there's probably general agreement that the system has worked fairly well in
spite of its trust in the integrity of the individual. Even though
there is some competition, they've been good about evaluating the
situation as honestly, fairly, and scientifically as they can. I'm
fairly well convinced that it's true. I'd like Paul Bianchi to
speak to this.

DR. BIANCHI: I certainly would agree with that. I think the
peer-review system at NIH has worked out very well. It's one of
the main things we're concerned with at NIH. Believe me, when you
serve on a study section, you're very conscious of your obligation
to NIH. I think this is one of the key points—that NIH is repre-
sentative of society as a whole, and through the peer-group reviews. NIH deliberately sets up a peer-review group. They go
outside their own institution and gather people from various segments of academic organizations. When one looks at a grant
proposal, one does a very thorough job of it, both in regard to
its design and with regard to the developments in the field—that
is, how important the particular project is. Is it something worth
supporting because the man has imagination and can push it forward?
In the pharmacology-study section we try to get balance in regard
to the experts in the field that are particularly involved. We
achieve interaction, a sort of balance that one needs when one
wants a "refereed" product.

I think this is what Dr. DeFelice is trying to achieve. But
he's achieving it through a private organization, which is always
faced with the problem raised by the speaker from Hoffman-LaRoche.
If you want a refereed decision, Dr. DeFelice should not be
supported by private organizations, but by the government or by
society as a whole. We are too much concerned with looking for
support either from private individuals or organizations, and yet
there's the collective responsibility with respect to this program.
The problem we're concerned with right now is how to achieve a

collective responsibility for what these drugs are doing in terms
of their benefit to society, and this is where the cultural lag
exists. There is no mechanism to achieve this collective responsibility. And this is one area where we do need this type of
responsibility. I'm afraid I don't see it on the horizon as yet.

DR. DeFELICE: I agree and I disagree. What I'm saying is
that we need a system that has all these components in it. I agree
with you. There is no public policy kind of mechanism in the
country. Perhaps the National Academy of Science should do it.
It's not, however, on the horizon. In the meantime, what do you
do? Sit back and wait for somebody to study prostaglandins? How
long are we going to wait? So what I'm saying is that you have to
get something moving and it's time for this kind of organization to
get moving. But never let it be said that a government institution
is not without vested interests. I repeat, never let it be said.
Look at the Food and Drug Administration. Look at what happened
to the NIH. Suddenly it put together new ethical guidelines for
the conduct of clinical trials as if to say it was negligent
before, which it really wasn't. There are mistakes in any system.
If a mistake occurs, do you change the system? Do you destroy
motherhood because of the batteredchild syndrome? I think that by
the very fact that decision making has "opened up" one cannot fool
the experts or the government. I can't, as the head of a private
organization, say a drug is good when it's not. There's too much
expertise out there. I'm almost forced to be objective, because I
will be found out if I'm not. One lousy report from me and I lose
my business. So I have to be honest by the nature of our present
values. So I think there are built-in balances to vested interests
today.

DR. PALMER: Gil McMahon has some questions or comments to make.

DR. McMAHON: Just a comment or two. I think company monitors
often have too much to do. Company physicians have responsibility
for several drugs in several different phases. In the past few

years they've had their jobs lightened a little bit by research
associates and paramedical people around them, and all this is
helpful. He's after the truth about his drug, both good and bad
effects. I think good data speaks for itself. Whether it comes
from Japan or Columbia or the U.S. isn't so critical to me. I
think good research and solid data speaks for itself. But personal
monitoring of data, wherever it is generated, is a necessary
function of company monitors.

DR. PALMER: We have a couple of drug monitors in the audience.
Would they agree with that statement that they have too much to do?

DR. MAZLEN: A qualified "Yes" would be my answer. From past
personal experience I would say the major problem is that top
administrators in the pharmaceutical industry are of a very non-
homogeneous background. Unfortunately, some decisions requiring a
significant clinical medical experience are made by persons of
diverse, nonmedical backgrounds. Due to the intrusion of misinfor-
mation, or of parochialism, these decisions may complicate the
trajectory of any development rather than simplify it.

Regarding monitor overloading, I would say that the individual
drug studies' monitor, usually a physician or a Ph.D., is becoming
more and more pivotal to successful new development. There is a
pressing need for the overall ethical pharmaceutical industry to
recognize the monitor's key role and to upgrade his professional
status as well as to provide for his or her continuing education in
clinical pharmacology and therapeutics. Today, in a general sense,
the drug monitor frequently is used as a means to an end rather than
as a means to achieve quality. In this respect, a monitor is often
overloaded by dint of the erroneous policy judgment, rampant in our
society, that quantity is identical to quality. Of course, the
patient is the final court in which the issue is to be settled.
Perhaps, with the advent of the age of consumerism, the public will
begin to demand an upgraded quality in drug development which drug
monitors are in a position to help achieve.

Also, I have a question for Dr. Clyde. Dr. Clyde, is there
any real basis to the current dogmatic cut-off value of the P value
of 0.05? If so, what is the proper place in clinical statistical
methods for statistical trends?

DR. CLYDE: If you have a study with a very small number of
patients, it's very difficult to get a P value as small as .05,
even with a massive difference. So in early Phase I studies, where
you may be trying to decide whether to drop the drug completely as
being unpromising, or whether to continue and spend more money on
research and get more cases, I would accept something larger than a
P value of .05 as a guide to further action. Now, I don't think
that the FDA is going to approve the drug if it cannot reach the
level of significance. But I think in the early stages you're
faced with a different decision. A company or an investigator is
faced with a decision whether to continue studying this drug or
some other drug. We're all in drug screening, whether we want to
be or not. Any company or any investigator wishes to pick a winner
early in the game. Since it's very difficult to get the .05 level
with just 10 patients, say, at that point I would pick something
like the .10 level or the .15 level as a guide to action. Suppose
I have the resources to pursue one drug and I have three possibilities. If one of the possibilities gives me something at the 15%
level in 10 patients, and the other two give me something at the
50% level, I would put my money on the 15% one. It's not conclusive; I know I'm not going to get it approved with 10 patients, but
it looks like that's the one which will lead to something.

Since the P value you can obtain does depend on the number of
patients, it works the other way, too. With 1,000 patients, it's
very easy to get a P value of .05. In fact, I'd say if you studied
1,000 patients, you'd better get something more significant than
.05 because that doesn't look so good anymore. I'll bet the FDA
wouldn't approve a drug that was studied on 1,000 patients with a
P value of .05; they would say this is such a negligible difference
with 1,000 patients, it's not worth arguing about. I'd raise my

sights as I went along. In the early stages, I'd accept a P value
that was not as significant as .05; in the final stages, we practically always see P values much more significant than .05.

Also, I think that the seriousness of the results must be
taken into account. If I can use an analogy, I might bet on a
horse if the P value of that horse winning was .15, the 15% level.
I wouldn't fly in an airplane if I thought the P value of my
getting killed was .15. It depends on the seriousness; when you're
talking about very serious effects of drugs, I think everyone would
want to be a little more sure than a P value of .15. What's good
enough in one situation is not good enough in another.

DR. DeFELICE: Speaking of statisticians, the one weakness in
our peer-group review, and I thought it was going to be our unequi-
vocal strength, was the addition of a statistician to it. I'll
tell you why. It's an intriguing situation. They're becoming as
powerful as the lawyers in the Food and Drug Administration. We
look at combinations, let's say in the gut. We use subjective
scales for our data. What has happened is the clinicians, and
even the Ph.D.'s who are supposed to know something about data,
withdraw as the statistician speaks about one tail or two tails.
Deliberations are thereby based upon the statistical interpretation
of that one member of the peer group, to which the other members
can't offer input. I'm not so sure that that man is right. So
we're thinking now of peering the statistician, perhaps two statisticians, one being removed from the peer group process. I don't
know how to handle this problem. Could you comment on this?

DR. CLYDE: As in every field, there are good statisticians
and there are bad statisticians. I think the best thing is to try
to get one good one. But it's a little hard sometimes to tell
whether you have a good one or a bad one, so I suppose there is
safety in numbers. Get two of them and hope that at least one of
them will give you good advice.

DR. HAGANS: I would like to offer just a brief minority point
of view about the P value for the applied man who's doing his

experiment to arrive at an answer. I believe there's really very
little sense to calculating a P value for interpretation unless
that experiment has been planned with the consideration of alpha
and beta risks and so on, unless there's been planning in the first
place, unless the kind of difference that's meaningful to the
applied person has been predefined, and unless sample size and the
consideration of power in the interpretation of that test has gone
into the planning and the execution of that experiment. Now, most
statisticians often won't tell you this because if they did,
roughly 70% of the tests that they do wouldn't be done; because
that kind of planning still doesn't go into most of the clinical
experimental work that's done. It's still a woefully small part
of it, which is kind of a testimony to the newness of statistics
and, as of this time, their failure to be thoroughly successful or
interested in being interdigitated into the planning phases of
clinical experimental work. But indeed, if you get a little bit
philosophical about this, although it may have a lot of mathematical interest and so on, if you simply do an experiment and do a
test and get a probability statement and then turn around and ask
if the difference observed is of any meaning and if it is then I'll
pay attention to it, and if it isn't....it's kind of illogical
reasoning really. There are these two different attitudes among
statisticians about the probability statement, I simply wanted to
represent this minority attitude, which I believe is growing.

DR. PALMER: I don't mean to be critical, but while you were
talking, Dr. McMahon pointed out that one of the difficulties is
that statisticians will all of a sudden mention a term that just
absolutely throws you off into space; dissociates one neurone from
another. That happened to me just now when you mentioned alpha
and beta risk factors. So I thought that I was pretty stupid,
until I asked Dr. McMahon and Dr. Cohen if they knew what they were
and they didn't know either.

DR. HAGANS: Well, I didn't mean to pull that kind of thing,
but I think all that does, Roger, is reflect to me the lack of

adequate communication between the fields of statistics and clinical research. The classical statistician tends to blame this all
on the clinical researcher. But as a matter of fact it's kind of
a 50:50 guilt situation. There is an awful lot of need in this
direction, but I think the trends are in the right direction. Ten
years ago there were about 10 statistical departments in the
roughly 100 medical schools that existed. Today there are something like 60 or 70. You know, the trend is in the right direction.
Intercommunication is going on better than it was, but it still is
nowhere where it ought to be. The result of this, in my personal
judgment, is that there's so much misapplication of statistical
techniques today that I'm scared it is going to give the whole
field a bad name. I really mean it, the baby is in danger of being
thrown out with the bathwater. It is a growing concern, and I
understand the hostility of the researcher. I also at times understand the hostility of the statistician. There's some justification
on both sides. The chief problem really is a problem of communication.

   Dr. Stanley Schor has said, "It is very difficult for the
statistician to scale the heights belonging to the medical investigators, and just as difficult for the medical investigator to
ascend the hill of the statistician. There must be a middle
ground—a plain between the two mountains; a place to which both
statisticians and medical investigators can lower themselves so
that they may fight on even terms." Fortunately, such plains do
exist today, but they are unfortunately not yet densely populated.
Therein lies a great deal of the present trouble.

   There's one small point that I want to raise and then I'll
quit. It's not related to what we were talking about. There's an
area in early clinical research where, as far as I know, there's no
statistical application possible, and yet it's an area, in my
opinion, that in our present state of the art has to exist. And
you sort of let the cat out of the bag when you said you give a
very small dose the first time in man before you do anything else.

What I'm trying to say is that there has to be a little early pilot
human experimental work in a nonstructured, perfectly free design
activity to a certain level of background experience before one can
even intelligently design the first controlled experiment. Without
it you're working in so much of a vacuum that you might as well
pack up and go home. Maybe some day our abilities and our techniques will get developed to where these two will meet. But they
don't meet at all right now. I have seen several articles recently
in the surgical literature where they're making the claim that, in
a new surgical technique in controlled trial, ramdomization should
occur from the very first operation—which to me is utter nonsense.
By translating it back to medicine (and there are similarities as
well as differences), this would say that your first small human
dose (which you know, except for anaphylaxis, isn't going to be
measurable in terms of any sort of response) would be put into the
randomization. This is utter nonsense. There isn't any statistical technique that I'm aware of that would handle this sort of
thing. I believe that all the worthwhile clinical investigators
that I know do early pilot studies. It's sort of like masturbation;
it's apparently something most everybody does but they don't talk
about it. It seems to be a bad sort of thing to talk about. It
shouldn't be.

I think we're coming to a real problem here, because the
rational as well as the irrational statistical influence is so
strong today that it's likely to get itself superimposed upon this
area of activity. The potential danger is far greater than any
possible reward at our present state. I think that it is a problem
that is just around the corner. The day may come when such pilot
work will be forbidden.

One final thought along that line is that I think we ought to
start thinking that the problem with doing uncontrolled pilot work
is two-fold. The enthusiastic investigator (and if he's an investigator he's enthusiastic, it's the nature of the beast) tends to
carry on pilot work too long. So first thing you know he's got 250

people in the pilot study and he's now convinced that the thing works. He's now got himself into an ethical quandry: can he do a controlled clinical trial when he knows it works? There's some place between this early experience and going too far that needs definition. I believe it could be defined if we'd focus on the problem. I don't think we've focused on that problem or given it proper thought at the present time.

DR. PALMER: To do the free kind of unstructured research that Dr. Hagans is talking about with human beings is, as I understand it, legally impossible, at least with the human-use committee. It is done, there's no question about it. It's done on each other, and nobody likes to talk about it. But if you do it and if something does happen, you're going to be in serious trouble. So you're really being hampered today in doing the Bill Harrington type of experiment where he injected stuff into himself to find out what really happened. Those types of experiments are virtually impossible to do. The human-use committee must approve any self- administration of any kind of a test drug. Even if you want to do it in the privacy of your own home, it has to go through the human-use committee. So you're really hampering this free form of investigation. Are there any comments from the audience?

DR. DICKSTEIN: This is not apropos to the past discussion except we still haven't had a definition of alpha and beta error. For practical purposes beta is perhaps of more concern to pharmaceutical organizations. Alpha is the chance that the drug will be proved effective but is ineffective; beta is the probability that in the light of the experimental evidence the drug will be proved to be ineffective but is really effective.

I'd like to pose a question to the panel. This has been touched on in past discussions, but I'd like to see if, based on pharmacological considerations rather than toxicological constraints, the panel can offer some advice as to selecting the initial dose in dose ranging in Phase I, and secondly, if the logical sequence of higher doses in dose ranging can be chosen.

DR. PALMER: I think it's just a guess. We try to shoot as
low as we possibly can, and I don't know of any kind of a scheme.
What we try to do is take one-tenth of the minimal effective dose
in the most sensitive species; minimal effective, not minimal
toxic or LD 50, because with LD 50s, as anybody will point out, you
have to know the shape of the curve. LD 50 per se isn't very
helpful. So we take about one-tenth of the minimal effective dose
as our first dose and we try to have the most sensitive measurements
that we can. Then we go up in an empirical increase, usually
doubling until we have an effect. Other people have other ideas.
Steve, you must have some thoughts on this.

DR. DeFELICE: When I was at Walter Reed there was a special
subcommittee which I headed on how to choose the first dose. I
spent two years reading about this subject. The conclusion is that
the best way to do this is to use what Dr. DiPalma calls "the
eyeballing method." You have to know how to look at all the data.
For example, the LD 50 doesn't tell you much. I don't know of any
correlation between LD 50 and people which one can hang one's hat
on. I don't know why it's done except to choose a dose for
subacute and chronic animal studies. I keep hearing it at meetings
as a parameter for the first dose in man. It's absurd. It's your
subacute toxicity and chronic toxicity dosing that gives you a
better indication of your first human dose.

Let's say your minimum toxic dose in subacute studies causes
weight loss with compound A and myocardial necrosis with compound
B. These both occur at 1 mg/kg. Would you use the same percentage
of both compounds as the initial dose in man? In other words, you
can't just give a figure. I heard someone say the other day that
for Phase II studies you take one-fourth of the dose in Phase I;
that's crazy. Generally speaking, but not always, one should use a
dose for Phase II studies that borders around the maximum tolerated
dose. If this dose shows no activity in man then you probably don't
have a drug, and you don't have to worry if your dose was too low.
But given the fact that we studied this for two years, we came up

with no rule of thumb. And it's just a matter that somebody has to know data—and have a smell for the whole picture. You must consider the nature of toxicity; what is known about the compound, etc. Then we choose a dose which is absurdly low as a first dose. This is what a clinical drug developer should be able to do.

DR. PALMER: I agree, because I feel that before we do a Phase I study we should get a hold of some of the material to allow those who are actually going to perform the investigation to use it in animals and get a feeling for the toxicity and for the minimal effect, rather than the LD 50. The example in question was one drug where the first effect that we saw in an animal was the widening of the QRS complex. That fit very well with its mode of action, so that's the first effect that we're going to look for. So we took one-tenth of the minimal effective dose in the most sensitive species, which was the dog. I agree that you have to get a feeling for the data by working with the compound yourself and have the resources of the laboratory and animals to do it. Gil, you must have some feeling about this.

DR. McMAHON: I'd like to tell Harvey that what I like in a protocol is sort of a different aspect. I like to have "room to move" in an early protocol. I like to start, of course, with a small dose that doesn't work; we expect that. But I am frustrated when you have to give the drug at a ceiling dose in the protocol, and you still have not reached efficacy or toxicity. I think it's a tragedy that you have to go back to the drawing boards with such a drug. I think you should be permitted to go on. I hate to be "boxed in," and I realize it isn't usually the company monitor's fault.

DR. PALMER: But it's difficult to tell whether you're having an effect or not. Let me give you an example. We took a compound with which we have been working, and we were pushing the dose and not getting an effect. Yet we knew we should be getting an effect on either heart rate or some autonomic function. When we recorded

the preejection period, we would see a nice shortening effect on
the preejection period before there was any effect on heart rate.
So if you have a sensitive measuring device you sometimes can pick
it up, unless you're working with crude things like heart rate and
blood pressure. With a cardiovascular drug you can have more
sensitive techniques like the preejection period.

DR. McMAHON: And the people who are giving phenobarbital were
not measuring P450 liver microsomal enzymes in 1898. I would agree
that the ejection times are a more sophisticated parameter which a
lot of investigators may not be measuring in Phase I, but I suggest
that they too will be regarded as primitive 50 years from now. So
all I say is you measure as much as you can and your main concern
is safety of the patient, as always. But you don't abandon the
drug if you don't see anything.

DR. DeFELICE: What Dr. McMahon said is an important issue of
the day—dosing and how you get there. Take the L-dopa story. I
think controlled studies data showed it not to work. Cotzias raised
the dose and it worked. You have to push dose under appropriate
circumstances. Because of the new moralism we're placing a lid on
appropriate dosing for Phase II by limiting dosing in Phase I. And
yet no one is saying anything. It's incredible that we're probably
evaluating dose levels in man which are not sufficient. And even
if the patient is fully informed and willing to take higher dosing,
he cannot. What, may I ask, is volunteering all about?

QUESTION FROM THE FLOOR: When do you abandon a drug?

DR. DeFELICE: The question was "when do I abandon a drug?"
Many times it is wise to place drugs to rest. Most drugs don't
make it to the market place. Yet before the burial much can be
learned. I think it's a very successful experiment when you've
given a drug to six people with gout in Phase I and you know that
it's uricosuric and you know it caused 4 out of 6 people to have
significant hepatic enzyme abnormalities; particularly when you
know it's effective in relieving the inflammation of gout. I think

that's a productive experiment despite the fact that the drug is
abandoned. You've buried the product but you've really stimulated
research into that series of compounds.

The answer to the question of "when to abandon?" is based on
the concept of risk-benefit; a concept that is quite flexible
depending on the vested interest. In sum, there is no specific
answer to the question.

DR. PALMER: Any further questions or comments from the panel?
We'll close then. I think it's been a successful discussion. We
haven't answered any questions at all. I think we've come full
circle, because last year in discussing drug development we came to
the conclusion that there ought to be some sort of an outside
refereeing agency, and it was brought up again whether it ought to
be private or government. And the suggestion was made last year
that it be a government agency that would answer generic questions
such as we posed today. This was a proposal of Jerry Levine of a
clinical pharmacology service center as a division of HEW. And
that idea is still alive and maybe some day will come true, I don't
know. I don't think it would put you out of business, Steve.

INDEX

A

Acetylcholine, 162–163, 221, 223
ACTH, 96, 103, 120, 190, 196, 200
Action potential, 134, 138–139, 164, 166, 168, 175, 177–178
Actomyosin, 155, 165
Adenylate cyclase, 83–84, 86–88, 90, 93–97, 99–106, 200
Adenylate cyclase system, prostaglandin sensitive, 109
Alkylating agents, 51
Alpha-adrenergic blockers, 120
American Society of Pharmacology, 2
Amidephrine, 126
Aminoglycoside antibiotic, 38, 40
Aminopyrene, 49
Amsler grid testing, 76
Angiotensin, 22, 164–165
Antihypertensives, 161
Antispermatogenic activity, 11
Aorta, rabbit, 167
Aortic strips, 164
Arachidonic acid, 189, 209, 213, 217
Aspirin, 47, 228
ATP, 83, 94, 98, 102, 107–110, 113, 139, 152–153, 155–157, 180
Audiograms, 44
AVP, 108–110, 112–113

B

Badrenergic agents, 161
Badrenergic blockers, 87, 89–90, 120, 126, 130
Badrenergic receptors, 89, 120–121, 128, 130
Benefit-risk ratio, 16, 24, 28, 255
Biostatisticians, 22
Bladder cancer, 50–52
Blood dyscrasia, 18

C

Caffeine, 136–138, 141, 143, 147–149
Calcium, 133–134, 139, 143–145, 147, 151–157, 162, 165–169, 173–180
Calcium pump, 153
Carcinogenicity, 11, 51
Carcinogenisis, chemical, 47, 49–52
Cardiac muscle, 168, 170, 174, 180
Cataractogenisis, 69–72
Cataracts, 69–72
Catecholamines, 83, 85, 89, 120–123, 125, 175–176, 207, 221
Chloramphenicol, 18, 31, 49, 72–74
Chloroquine, 73–77
Chlorpromazine, 50
Chlortetracycline, 151–153
Clinical pharmacologists, 3, 19
Clinical Resources, Inc., 239
Clyde mood scale, 233
Cocaine, 31
Cochlea, 32, 34, 37, 43
Cochlear potential, 33–35, 37, 41–44
Colebrine, 128
Colon cancer, 52
Color vision, 67
Color vision testing, 76